C0-BXA-818

Library of
Davidson College

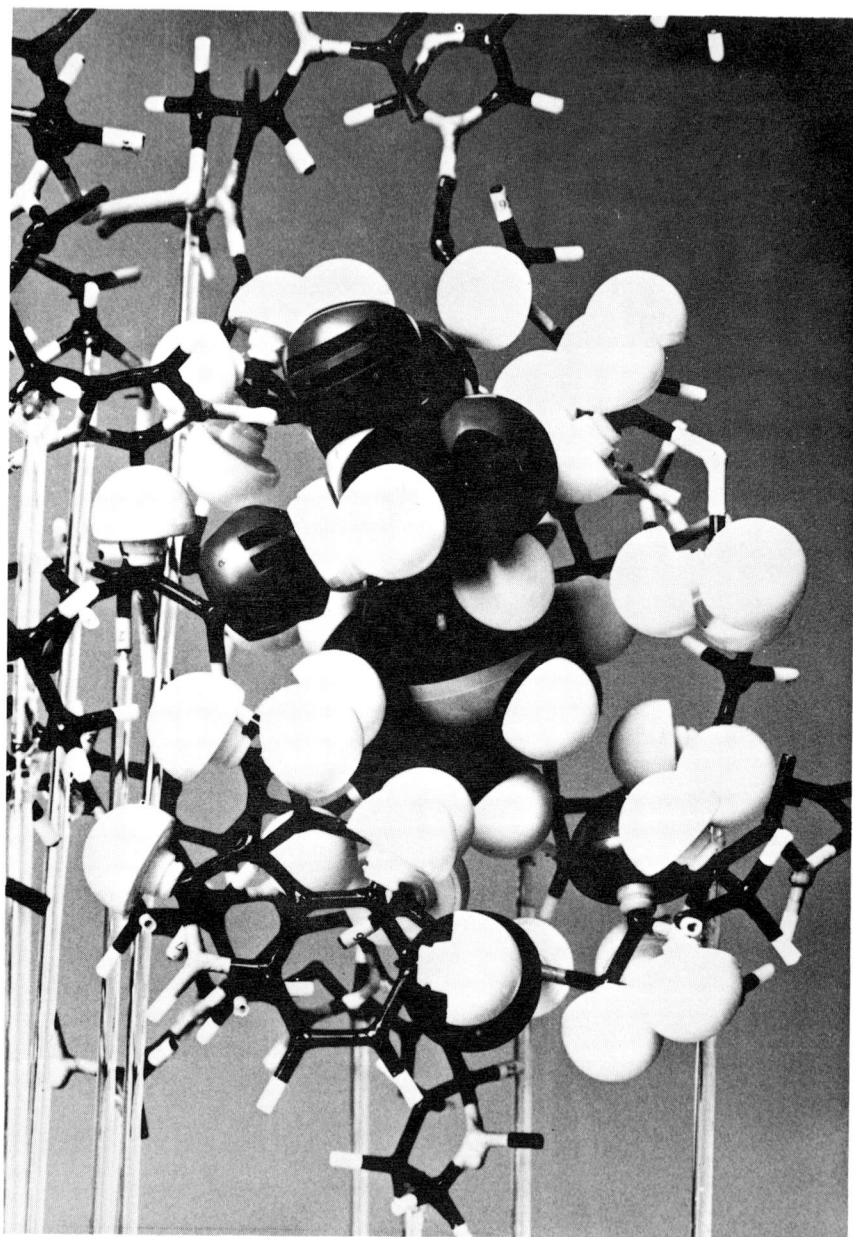

Substrate in Specificity Cavity: Model for Drug-Receptor Interaction
(For explanation see 167).

HOW MODERN MEDICINES ARE DISCOVERED

Edited By
FRANK H. CLARKE, Ph.D.

FUTURA
PUBLISHING COMPANY
1973

615.1

C 597R

Copyright © 1973
Futura Publishing Company, Inc.

Published by
Futura Publishing Company, Inc.
295 Main Street
Mount Kisco, New York 10549

L.C.#: 73-80696
ISBN#: 0-87993-027-6

All rights reserved. 75-4218
No part of this book may be translated or reproduced in
any form without the written permission of the publisher.

CONTENTS

There has been no easy road leading to the discovery of modern medicines. This is reflected by the expenditure of nearly 4.4 billion dollars by American pharmaceutical companies for research and development during the period from 1962–71. Not included in this figure are the millions of dollars spent annually for medicinal research programs at American universities and research institutes. During this 10-year period, only 170 newly synthesized drugs were marketed.

One of the key scientists involved in drug discovery is the medicinal chemist, for it is he or she who usually initiates the chain of events which culminates in the development of a new medicinal agent. Sometimes hundreds of compounds are prepared in a single laboratory before a promising potential drug is uncovered, and even then the odds are great that it will not survive the vigorous battery of animal toxicity studies and clinical testing.

Although the past record of success in the search for new medicines is considerably less than one can expect at a gambling casino, future prospects look more promising because medicinal chemists are now employing principles of drug design unknown a decade ago. Indeed, books and articles on this subject are now widely read, and within the near future these principles will be used routinely for optimizing the efficiency of drug discovery.

The authors of this book are all engaged in medicinal research and hence are well qualified to describe the history and hurdles of their profession. They have provided lucid descriptions, using selected examples to ensure that the reader gains a broad appreciation of drug discovery from the viewpoint of the medicinal chemist. This book is addressed principally to those with some knowledge of biology and chemistry who wish to obtain a broad overview on this topic. Students who are interested in pursuing graduate studies in medicinal research and in the medical and allied professions will find it particularly valuable.

Professor Philip S. Portoghese
Department of Medicinal Chemistry
College of Pharmacy
University of Minnesota

PREFACE

In this book the story of the discovery of modern medicines has been told by medicinal researchers. No attempt has been made to present an entire picture of such research. Instead, a number of scientists in pharmaceutical research laboratories have drawn from their own experience, knowledge and expertise to write these chapters. Naturally, the authors have expressed their own views; others might have used different examples to illustrate particular areas of medicinal discovery. Many important subjects, such as research on the prostaglandins and the discovery of nonsteroidal anti-inflammatory agents are not covered. Nevertheless, the topics selected are illustrative, and we hope will provide the reader with an appreciation for the exciting moments that illuminate the long, enormously complex paths that lead to new agents to cure disease or to alleviate its symptoms.

This project originated with Dr. Gerald Laubach, now president of Pfizer Inc., in his former role as chairman of the Research Information Committee of the Pharmaceutical Manufacturers Association. It was Dr. Laubach's idea to describe significant advances that are being made by dedicated scientists in the pharmaceutical industry in a way that would be easily understood by science-oriented readers. Even for such readers a gap must be bridged when scientific matters are described. The scientist himself is often least prepared to accomplish this task. Still, this is what we have tried to do, and we hope that the frequent explanations of difficult terms will provide assistance. The use of structural formulas—the pictorial language of the medicinal chemist—is described in the Appendix. There is also discussion there of the names of drugs. Further assistance for the reader who wishes to delve deeper is provided by selections of Suggested Readings at the end of each chapter.

I wish to thank the Pharmaceuticals Division, CIBA-GEIGY Corporation for generous support throughout the course of this project. Special thanks are due to Shirly D. Brindle of the Drug Metabolism Sub-division for assistance with the illustrations of autoradiography in Chapter 8; to Dr. Karl Brunings, vice president, for many helpful discussions; to Craig Cooper of the Sub-division of Metabolic Diseases for photographs of the models in Chapter 3 and the illustrations of autoradiography in Chapter 8; to Franz Mohr of the Photography Department for assistance with a number of the photographs in Chapter 8—especially Figures 8, 9 and 10; to my secretary, Anne Porto, for typing and retyping parts of the manuscript and to Alex Valow of the Art Department for the structural formulas, many of the line drawings and the legends for the figures.

I wish to express my appreciation and thanks to William Cray, vice president, and Mary Halas, publications editor, of the Pharmaceutical Manufacturers Association for their excellent editorial revision of the manuscript, to Mr. Cray for making arrangements with the publisher; to Ms. Halas for preparation of the index; and to Dr. John Adams, PMA vice president, and C. Joseph Stetler, PMA president, for helping to make this project possible.

I also wish to acknowledge assistance during the early stages of this project from William E. Chace, W. C. Fernelius, Robert F. Gould, Dr. Robert Quinnel, John M. Sullivan and Robert E. Varnerin.

Sincere appreciation is expressed to the authors and publishers who graciously gave permission to use previously published illustrative material. Individual credits are acknowledged in the figure legends.

I am very much indebted to Dr. Bill Elpern and Dr. Ralph Vinegar for their critical reviews of the entire manuscript and to Dr. Donald Buyske for assistance with Chapter 8, to Bruce Collins with Chapters 1 and 3, to Dr. Richard Hinman with Chapter 1, and to Dr. Everette May and Dr. Albert Pohland for help with Chapter 3.

I wish to thank Dr. Gerald Laubach and the members of the Committee on Research Information and Professional Relations of the Pharmaceutical Manufacturers Association for their help and encouragement throughout this project.

Finally, I thank Steven Korn and Jacques Strauss of Futura Publishing Company for their advice and assistance in the final preparation of the manuscript.

Frank H. Clarke, PhD
Pharmaceuticals   Division,
CIBA-GEIGY Corporation

CHAPTER 1

How Modern Medicines Are Discovered

Frank H. Clarke

In his poem about the fairy prince who found the sleeping beauty, Tennyson wrote, "This proverb flashes thro' his head, 'The many fail, the one succeeds." The same thought applies to the modern medicinal researcher who contemplates the many compounds identified in the course of finding one that does work. Of the thousands of new compounds prepared and evaluated each year only a handful ever find actual use in patients.

Something very special is required to succeed. This is one of the reasons why the search for new medicines is important and challenging. The goal of medicinal researchers is nothing short of the control of disease. They must apply advances in many branches of modern scientific research to the problem of correcting abnormal function in the chemistry of living systems. Successful drug research requires an interdisciplinary approach involving clinicians, biologists, chemists and mathematicians—a unique effort with few parallels in the world of science.

A Team To Meet the Challenge

True, a multidisciplinary approach among human endeavors is not unique. The concepts of "team" and "teamwork" in American football provide an apt analogy to illustrate the strategies and cooperation essential in modern medicinal research. In football today all players are specialists—linebackers, cornerbacks, wide receivers, kickers, tactician quarterbacks, strategist coaches and so on. All these team members have to understand each other. Well executed plays depend on each specialist making his contribution to the yardage gain, the touchdown or the field goal. The fact that many of the plays (plans) don't turn out as

1

expected has not caused any of the winning teams to discard the planned approach. Nonetheless, many games are won by the unexpected pass interception, recovered fumble or blocked kick. The advantage seems to accrue to the best prepared team, its players combining skill and individual initiative to seize opportunity. So it is with drug research.

The Initial Concept

How do we begin to discover a new chemical compound that will be a useful therapeutic agent? When modern molecular biology comes of age, we might hope to be able to design new compounds at the molecular level from an understanding of the causes of disease and of the properties of molecules. Although later chapters will document that science is making dramatic progress, coming ever closer to this goal; it has not yet been reached.

If medications cannot yet be tailored to meet therapeutic requirements, what are the origins of ideas that lead to their discovery? Later we shall examine this question in some detail, but for the moment let's point to some of the many possible approaches.

Many medicines prescribed today are natural products. Their use can be traced back to the early pages of history. One such drug is morphine. We still lack a rational theory to explain drug action in analgesia (pain alleviation). The most fruitful approach has been to modify the drug that works—morphine—and attempt to prepare a related compound that retains the analgesic properties without the undesirable side effects.

Important examples of the successful modification of natural products are found among the antibiotics. The story of the tetracyclines and penicillins offers exciting testimony to the power of this approach.

Other drugs are discovered as a result of serendipity (the discovery of an object not searched for) in pharmacology and the clinic. A rational approach to drug discovery with sulfonamide antibiotics—the antimetabolite concept—led to clinical testing of likely prospects. One of these showed dramatic activity, not in the area expected, but as a diuretic. Alert biologists followed up this lead and soon opened a whole new area of drug research. Another example of serendipity in the clinic was the discovery that certain of the antihistamines are potent depressants of the central nervous system. This approach to tranquilizers has been followed by the more sophisticated design of compounds with particular effects on the biochemistry of the brain. As biologists and biochemists became intrigued by the possibility that the excessive action of certain enzymes was responsible for mental disease, a new avenue appeared in the search for drugs that affect the central nervous system. This quest led to compounds designed to inhibit the enzymes believed responsible for abnormal brain function.

The discovery of a new drug may have its origin in the modification of a natural product that has a desired therapeutic effect or, on the other hand, in rational concepts of the nature of disease and of the metabolic fate of a therapeutic agent. Between these two extremes lies the area of research based on the new lead. A lead is the often accidental discovery that a compound has a desired activity in an animal or in man. To be prepared for unusual discoveries in scientific research, we must continue testing the biological effects of compounds in whole animals.

Screening

Before a new drug is tested in man, the researcher must have some logical basis for assuming that it will have the desired activity. The most convenient animals for initial (screening) tests are usually small rodents, such as mice and rats, but small dogs and monkeys often are used. The smaller animals are economical and are relatively easy to handle. In one test for analgesia, a mouse is treated with the test compound and its tail is then exposed to the heat of an infrared lamp. The tail flicks when the mouse feels pain. The time required for the mouse to react is recorded as the latency period for the test compound. This simple model for pain works well in evaluating potential analgesics.

On the other hand sophisticated models of disease have been developed by pharmacologists to test potential new medicines. Some of these require great skill and ingenuity. In the search for drugs to treat mental diseases, many laboratories have used procedures in which animals learn to escape an electric shock or to get food by pressing a lever. High blood pressure has been produced in dogs and rats, and the techniques have been applied to the discovery of agents that lower blood pressure.

The testing of potential drugs for activity against bacterial cultures is widely known, and discovery of the antibiotics in this manner is one of the great milestones in the history of drug therapy. Until modern times, the dearth of knowledge about the nature of viruses has severely handicapped progress in this area, but now development of such tests for antiviral activity is well advanced. As the molecular structures of viruses become known, their method of attack on host cells is better understood. Viruses can reproduce only within the host cell, making the problem still difficult, but the door has been opened to usher in the antiviral era.

Modern approaches to controlling cardiovascular and central nervous system diseases involve new concepts of biochemical changes. Later chapters in this book discuss biochemical screening procedures used in the search for inhibitors of specific enzymes that are involved in the synthesis or degradation of a hormone.

Whole new areas of research are emerging as we map molecular structures of enzymes and learn details of their mechanisms. Consider the potential for the future when the secrets of the body's defenses—the immune phenomena—are understood and controlled!

Evaluation

A new lead discovered in a biological screen sets in motion a train of events. The pharmacologist and the biochemist examine the behavior of the new compound in sophisticated tests, and the chemist evaluates the novelty of the discovery in terms of chemical structure. Larger amounts of the new compound are prepared for detailed toxicity studies in animals, and arrangements are made to study the potential new drug in man.

As the testing gathers momentum, more and more scientists become involved, each with an important part to play in the discovery procedure. These experts continually evaluate the drug during this period against initial expectations.

In the beginning stages of the process, it is the biologist who asks the questions. He repeats the original test at the same dose, at higher and at lower doses, in other species or by other routes of administration—orally, intraperitoneally, subcutaneously, intravenously. Other models for the disease may be selected as the testing proceeds.

If more extensive studies support the original test results, the biological researcher examines the test compound for its potential to cause severe toxicity. Acute toxicity is first established—the single dose required to cause death in 50 percent of the animals tested. Occasionally a new compound that appears to be potentially useful in early tests turns out to be too toxic. A successful drug usually must have a high therapeutic ratio: That is, the toxic dose must be much greater than the dose required for therapy.

In these early tests, we look especially for possible side effects. Does the animal have tremors? Does necrosis (destruction of tissue) occur at the site of injection? Is the animal depressed or stimulated?

While the pharmacologist confirms and extends his tests for useful activity of the new compound, the biochemist may determine its effect on enzyme systems or hormones, hoping to discover its mechanism of action or to detect potential side effects. In some cases, he may try the new compound on biochemical models of the disease to see how it compares with standard drugs.

The biochemist also studies the absorption of the new compound into the blood stream from the gastrointestinal tract. Many new medicines must be made available in an oral tablet or capsule form. To be effective, they must be absorbed into the blood stream from the stomach or the intestine. The concentration of a drug in the blood stream is particularly important: The drug level in the blood must be high enough to exert a therapeutic effect at the target organ, and the drug must remain in the blood stream long enough to sustain the beneficial effect.

Tissue studies indicate the concentrations of the candidate drug in various organs of the body. From these results and from studies of excretion of the compound in the urine or feces, we can learn whether it tends to accumulate in the body. This information is vital, especially if the new agent will be used on a long-term basis for a chronic illness. Such findings may advance efforts to improve dosage so as better to sustain drug levels in the blood and to prolong action.

The manner in which an animal handles the potential drug is also the object of extensive studies. More often than not the body has a mechanism that alters an invading compound to make it less toxic, more soluble and thus more easily eliminated in the urine. Even in early studies for which clinical trials are planned, it is important to determine the metabolic pattern in the animal species subject to the chronic toxicity studies. Later, when the drug is tested in man, its metabolic pattern again is observed and compared with that seen in the animals. Ideally, chronic toxicity studies should be carried out in an animal species whose metabolic pattern is close to that of man.

Sensitive methods of analysis, developed in many cases by natural product chemists, have been used to detect and characterize small amounts of metabolic products in biological fluids. Methods include spectroscopic techniques, such as infrared, ultraviolet, nuclear magnetic resonance and mass spectroscopy. Such analytical tools, coupled with powerful separation techniques such as thin-layer and vapor-phase chromatography, provide practical means for mapping metabolic patterns. It may not be necessary to isolate and identify each and every metabolite, but as the studies proceed it is important to obtain evidence that the species chosen for chronic toxicity studies is similar to the human being in the way it reacts to the new drug.

Chemistry

The new lead lures the chemist to the challenge of discovery. He designs each of his trial compounds to be active in the

disease model, but at the outset the prospect that any one of
these compounds would prove satisfactorily active and nontoxic
is only a fond hope. The request for more compound for further biological studies is often the first clue to approaching
success. The clue usually results in questions for the chemist:
Why this particular compound? How does the new lead compare with the standard test compound (which is often the medication now being sold)? How many compounds of this new
class are active? Is there a structure-activity pattern that will
lead to still further improvement? Scientists seek answers to a
variety of such questions as they pursue the new lead.

While researchers explore these scientific parameters, they
also consider the novelty and patentability of the discovery.
The United States' system of patent protection provides the
incentive for the vast expenditure of time and money necessary
if the lead is ever to mature into a marketable drug. When the
scope and limits of the discovery are clearly defined by chemical and biological studies, a patent application may be drafted
and filed.

When the biologist requires larger amounts of the compound
for his more extensive studies—especially of subchronic toxicity
in larger animals—the chemist supplies several kilograms of the
new substance. By this time, its synthesis assumes a new per-
spective. What was possible on a small scale in the laboratory
often becomes impractical and unsafe on a large scale. So process development begins. Specialists seek new synthetic approaches that will offer the advantages of safety on a larger scale
and that will be economically attractive. As new routes to synthesis of the compound unfold, new derivatives and related
compounds can be made from new and different intermediates.
Often new chemical reactions are discovered and old ones are
explored in a fresh light.

Later, as developmental chemists undertake large scale synthesis, analytical chemists study the physical properties of the
new compound in detail. They may have to develop new methods to detect small amounts of impurities that must be removed
or identified and studied biologically before any tests are carried out in man.

As the biochemist extends his studies to metabolism, he develops methods to detect trace amounts of the compound and

its metabolites in animal tissues. He may have to synthesize these metabolites for a positive identification. As we shall see in Chapter 8, the new substance may have to be labeled by radioactive carbon or tritium atoms in order to delineate metabolism.

Toxicology

When continued testing confirms and extends the initial impression that the compound possesses useful activity in animal models of the disease, researchers can make plans for testing in man. Prior to human subject testing, however, they must carry out extended toxicity studies in animals to determine, as nearly as possible, what dose will be safe in man. This is often difficult, because the compound's effect in man may not be the same as in animals.

Studies of acute toxicity in at least three or four species of animals and subchronic toxicity in at least two species of mammals help to overcome this problem. One of the species may be a rodent, but the other will be a nonrodent, usually a dog or a monkey. A subchronic project takes from two weeks to three months, and it is usually longer than the full course of the therapy proposed for man. The object of these studies is to find not only the highest no-effect dose but also the lowest dose at which some toxic manifestation appears. The first toxic symptoms in the animals provide a warning for clinicians to look for possible danger in man.

Doses of different magnitudes are usually given simultaneously to several groups of healthy animals, both male and female, in the same way the drug ultimately will be used in man. A control group of similar healthy animals live under the same conditions but receive no drug. During the entire experiment the investigators keep detailed records of observations on the health of the animals, noting especially any abnormalities. When the experiment is completed, they scrupulously examine the animals' internal organs for signs of toxicity. Every bit of data is carefully evaluated for safety to determine whether a recommendation should be made for testing in man.

It is important that the very compound examined in these toxicity studies be used in clinical trials. To be sure that this is the case, the formulation development chemist usually prepares a single batch of the compound. Some of the batch goes into animal testing, and pending the successful outcome of the toxicity experiment, some goes into human trials. At this stage, formulation development of the new medicine is often kept to a minimum, but when human efficacy is established, all the forms in which the drug may be given to man—capsules, pressed tablets, coated tablets and solutions for injections—come under consideration.

Clinical Pharmacology

Clinical investigators carry out initial tests of a potential new medication in man with great caution. Before they decide to begin a clinical trial, they review results of all the pharmacological and toxicological studies in animals. No absolute criteria apply in this evaluation of the preclinical phase. If animal studies have shown a high potential for toxicity, the investigators must weigh potential therapeutic values of the new agent against that of established products before deciding whether the benefits of the proposed clinical study justify the risk.

Both the sponsor of the potential drug and the Food and Drug Administration—a regulatory agency of the federal government—share the responsibility for assessing the adequacy of the animal data. The sponsor must submit to the FDA the detailed animal data from which he has concluded that he can conduct a clinical investigation with reasonable safety.

First studies in man are carried out by physician investigators who work with healthy individuals in a controlled situation to determine safety of the new medication. If safety requirements are met in these tests the new compound may be evaluated for efficacy. Well established specialist physicians working with patients seek to demonstrate an advantage over existing therapy. The advantage could be reduced side-effects, greater effectiveness in controlling the disease, or both. Relative potency, as determined by a comparison of the dosages required to achieve the same therapeutic effect, is not the most important criterion unless it is clear that increased potency (lower dose required) is associated with fewer or milder side effects.

New Drug Application

Introduction of a new medicine on the market culminates a long series of precise investigations, each phase longer, more complicated, and more costly than the one before. Every effort is made, of course, to find advantages of the new agent. It must do something that is not achieved with current drug therapy or it will have difficulty competing in the marketplace. It is important to know what is wrong with existing therapy—not only for the scientist anxious to demonstrate the advantages of the new discovery but also for those in market research who must estimate the medical potential of these advantages.

As clinical trials proceed, they involve large numbers of patients, and the scientists also compare the metabolic fate and pattern in man with those found previously in animals. Meanwhile, animal experiments continue to gather more data for assessing safety. The effect of the drug on the developing fetus of litter-bearing animals is studied before the potential new product may be administered to pregnant women or to women of childbearing age.

If these studies continue to demonstrate safety and efficacy in man, the pharmaceutical company collects and organizes all the voluminous data required for a new drug application. The Food and Drug Administration must approve the application before the new product can be prescribed by physicians. Such review may take many months, or even years, and the agency may request additional studies.

The requirements for safety and for demonstrable efficacy make the whole process of introducing a new product long, tedious, demanding and costly. It requires uncommon patience and a dogged capacity to surmount disappointment. But the goal is splendid—nothing short of a safer, more effective agent to alleviate and control disease. In the following chapters, we shall see how this goal has been approached in the past and how well it has been attained. And along the way, we shall provide a few glimpses of horizons expanding into the future.

Suggested Reading

Arnow, L. E. *Health in a Bottle.* Pennsylvania: J. B. Lippincott, 1970.

Cooley, D. G. *The Science Book of Modern Medicines.* New York: Franklin Watts, 1963.

deKruif, P. *Microbe Hunters.* New York: Pocket Books, 1943.

Dowling, H. F. *Medicines for Man.* New York: Alfred A. Knopf, 1970.

Rubin, A. A. *Search for New Drugs.* New York: Marcel Dekker, 1972.

Walker, N. *Medicine Makers.* New York: Hastings House Publishers, 1966.

CHAPTER 2

Natural Antibiotics

G. E. Mallett

Sir Alexander Fleming started it all in 1928, when he observed a mold growing on a plate of *Staphylococcus aureus*, a disease-causing (pathogenic) bacterium. Around the mold was a clear area where the staphylococcus did not grow. Fleming realized that the mold produced something that prevented growth of the pathogenic bacterium and that the same product of the mold might have the capacity to cure an infectious disease by preventing growth of bacterial parasites in infected hosts.

Fleming's insight was correct. As is now well known, the mold he happened on was *Penicillium notatum*, and the product was the storied antibiotic, penicillin—a medicine that has helped to cure millions of infections and to protect millions of lives.

Antibiotics are natural products produced by microorganisms, and they have the unique property of inhibiting the growth of other microorganisms. A multitude of infectious diseases resulting from growth of pathogenic bacteria in the human body have caused pain, disability and death since the beginning of time. By their ability to prevent such growth, antibiotics have become one of the most useful classes of drugs. In the years since World War II, antibiotics have reduced the death rate from infectious diseases dramatically.

The research launched by Fleming has been continued by scientists around the world. They have isolated and characterized hundreds of antibiotics, and have developed a few into useful medicines.

The search for new antibiotics persists because antibiotic therapy, for all its achievements, remains imperfect. There are still no completely satisfactory types for some infectious microorganisms. Infections caused by fungi and certain strains of *Pseudomonas* are difficult to control.

The Quest for New Antibiotics

Some antibiotics are quite effective against the target disease organisms but have drawbacks to their widespread use in human beings. For example, vancomycin effectively controls staphylococcal infections, but it must be administered intravenously. This method of administration is satisfactory for hospital patients but is not generally suitable for home use.

Finally, bacteria display a remarkable capacity to adapt to the environment and to survive. In the course of therapy an occasional bacterial cell is able to survive in the presence of the antibiotic. If this cell grows and multiplies, a population of resistant cells may emerge. For example, after the advent of penicillin therapy, strains of staphylococcus emerged with the ability to produce penicillinase. This enzyme, which destroys penicillin, renders these cells resistant to the antibiotic. Such resistant cells are more difficult to kill with the original drug, and an alternate mode of therapy (use of a different antibiotic) is indicated. Therefore, the search for new antibiotics to supplement those currently available continues.

The quest for a new antibiotic begins with a culture of a microorganism—perhaps from the molds, perhaps from a filamentous (threadlike) group of organisms, the genus *Streptomyces,* or perhaps from a newly discovered, unique group of microorganisms.

There is a sense of excitement at the beginning. The odds against finding an important new antibiotic are overwhelming. And yet, one can look at each new culture and say: "Is this the one? Will this culture produce a new antibiotic that will benefit thousands of patients?" To find the answer, researchers grow the culture in a nutrient broth solution, usually in a shaken flask. If the culture produces an antibiotic, some portion of it should be present in the broth.

Scientists have devised a simple technique to detect the presence of antibiotic in such cultures. They dip a little pad of filter paper into the broth to absorb some of the liquid and then lay it on an agar plate that has been seeded with a test organism (the target bacterium). Several different test plates may be used. On one, the test organism may be a strain of *Staphylococcus aureus.* This organism is included not only because it is a pathogen but also because it is useful in detecting antibacterial substances effective against other members of its class of pathogens known as gram-positive bacteria. (The terms *Gram positive* and *Gram negative* are convenient classifying terms based on staining reactions observed under the microscope.) On another plate, the test organism may be a strain of *E. coli*, both a pathogen itself and a detector of antibacterial substances effective against gram-negative pathogens. On still another plate, the test organism may be *Neurospora crassa*, a mold that detects antifungal activity.

The test plates are then incubated, permitting the test organism to grow until the surface becomes cloudy. However, if the pad contains an antibiotic, its presence is indicated by a clear zone around the pad. Something in the pad has diffused into the seeded agar and inhibited the growth of the test organism. (See Figure 1.) That something may be a new antibiotic and becomes the subject of further investigation.

Chromatographic Techniques

The unknown substance noticed in the primary detection system can now be defined only by its observed capability to inhibit the growth of a test organism, such as *Staphylococcus aureus.* Many antibiotics already discovered are able to do that much. Before proceeding with isolation and evaluation, we need to know whether the substance really is new or is an already known antibiotic. The primary tool for making this evaluation is the paper chromatogram. Different substances have characteristic ways of moving in given chromatographic systems. Thus, we can learn whether the substance is new or known by comparing its chromatographic mobility with that of the known antibiotics. The problem, however, is that at this stage we know

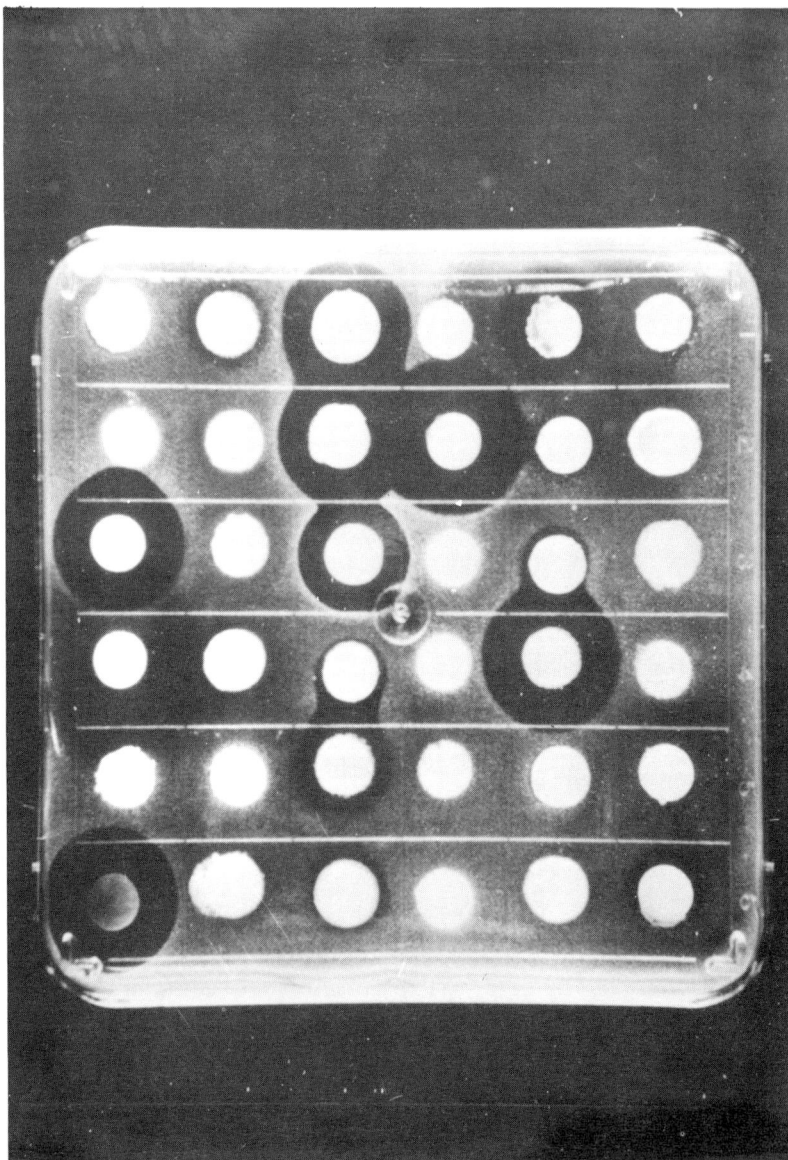

Figure 1. Zones of inhibition can be seen around some of the pads laid on this seeded agar plate. The zones indicate antibiotic activity. From "Bacteriologic Research Technics—Antibiotic Screening" by Gordon E. Mallett, *Tile and Till*, Vol. 53, No. 4 (December 1967), Eli Lilly and Company.

nothing about the chemistry of the new material, and detecting it on the chromatogram by ordinary chemical detection methods would be difficult.

One thing, though, is known about the substance: It inhibits the growth of staphylococcus, as do penicillin V, erythromycin, tylosin and certain other antibiotics. But if it is chemically different from the known antibiotics and is indeed new, it will move to a different spot on a paper chromatogram. Therefore, to put the unknown substance to the test, the producing culture is grown again and a fraction of a milliliter of the culture fluid is applied to a paper chromatogram. After the researcher has developed the chromatogram, removed it from the solvent system and dried it, he then lays it on a seeded agar plate similar to the one on which the activity was first discovered. Next he presses the chromatogram into intimate contact with the seeded agar, permitting the antibiotic to diffuse from the paper into the agar. Under incubation the test organism grows except in those spots where there is antibacterial activity. (See Figure 2.)

In this way the position of the substance on the chromatogram can be determined. In a sense, the chromatogram has given us, through its biological activity, the autograph of the antibiotic—hence the term *bioautograph*. Knowing the chromatographic mobility of the as yet unidentified substance, we can compare it with those of all known antibiotics.

Isolation and Evaluation

If the compound is indeed new, the excitement mounts. We have found a rare thing, a new antibiotic. But now the scientists must isolate and characterize the compound. To accomplish this task, the fermentation specialist must improve the yield, and the isolation chemist must separate it from all other substances that were present in the original broth or were produced by the growing microorganism along with the antibiotic.

The fermentation specialist studies the composition of the fermentation medium, the environmental factors (temperature, aeration rate, agitation) and the strain of the producing microorganism. He manipulates these factors in his attempts to optimize the yield.

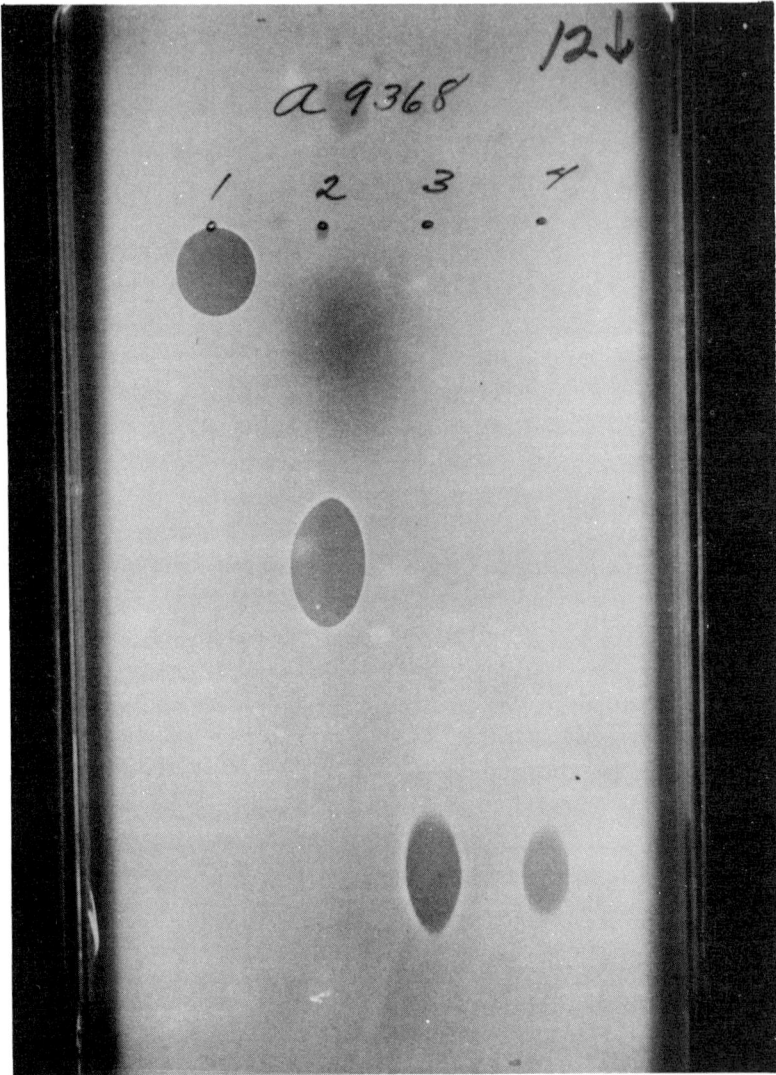

Figure 2. A bioautograph is made with a paper chromatogram. The zones of inhibition indicate the location of antibiotic activity, corresponding to the location of the antibiotic on the paper chromatogram. Lane 1, erythromycin A standard. Lane 2, erythromycin B. Lane 3, erythromycin C. Lane 4, Unknown compound, which moves as does erythromycin C and which may be erythromycin C. From "Bacteriologic Research Technics—Antibiotic Screening" by Gordon E. Mallett, *Tile and Till*, Vol. 53, No. 4 (December 1967), Eli Lilly and Company.

At the same time, the chemist studies separation techniques, such as precipitation, adsorption on carbon or ion exchange resins and solvent extraction—searching for ways to separate the desired antibiotic from the undesired remainder of the fermentation broth. He selects the useful techniques and arranges them in the preferred order to yield the desired compound in highest purity. Ultimately, he attempts to crystallize the new antibiotic.

During the fermentation and isolation program, the concentration of antibiotic in the fermentation or in the isolated fraction is measured by using a microbiological assay. Such assays typically involve quantitative measurement of the effect of the antibiotic on growth of the test organism. In one type of assay, the procedure described earlier for the detection of an antibiotic is standardized and quantified. These studies can establish a precise relationship between the diameter of the zones of inhibition and the concentration of antibiotic in the solution on the filter paper pad.

During the fermentation and isolation studies, the researchers take pains to assure that the fermentation is still producing the same new antibiotic. This they do by returning at frequent intervals to the paper chromatographic systems.

As the isolation work proceeds, investigations begin in the biology laboratories. The antibiotic, first detected because of its ability to inhibit a simple test organism, is tested against many test organisms that cause infective diseases. The test organisms include antibiotic-resistant strains.

A series of tests in animals supplement these *in vitro* investigations. For example, mice infected with the test organisms receive the new antibiotic, so that the course of the infection can be noted. These experiments establish the *in vivo* activity of the drug. Many antibiotics are active *in vitro* but are either inactivated or not absorbed in the body, and thus are not active *in vivo*.

Other vital information gathered through these animal experiments includes the preferred mode of administration (Is the drug active when taken orally or must it be administered by injection?) and the toxicity of the compound. Many new antibi-

otics, highly active *in vitro* but highly toxic *in vivo*, have caused
disappointments.

Developing the New Antibiotic

Obviously, an antibiotic that inhibits many clinically important strains and that is active *in vivo* without obvious toxicity
emerges as a potentially important new drug. But there is much
more research ahead. The organic chemist concerns himself with
the characterization of the compound—solubility, stability and
structure. All are important. Formulation chemists seek an appropriate, stable dosage form so that the drug is readily available in a form acceptable to patients.

Detailed studies on pharmacology and toxicology must be
made. The biochemist studies metabolism, tissue distribution
and the mode and rate of excretion. The pharmacologist inves-
tigates the impact of the antibiotic on cardiovascular, renal,
central nervous and other systems in the body. The toxicologist
examines the effects of high doses and of prolonged administration to several species of animals. His concerns include a
wide variety of indicators of toxic effects, including blood and
urine chemistry, tests for liver function, effects on reproductive
function and teratology (formation of malformed offspring).
These studies are a preliminary to administration of the compound to man. As explained in Chapter 1, such studies are done
to provide as much assurance as possible about safety and efficacy before testing in a human being.

When an investigational new drug exemption (IND) has been
approved, the drug is first administered by a trained physician
to carefully selected patients. Initially, these studies determine
human tolerance of the drug as well as appropriate dosage.

The first dose is only a small fraction of the amount believed
necessary for therapeutic activity. If no untoward symptoms
appear, the physician investigator cautiously increases the dose.
He monitors the concentrations of antibiotic in the patients'
blood after each increasing dose until it exceeds the concentration needed to inhibit growth of the infectious microorganism. He then administers the antibiotic at that dose level
and observes therapeutic effect and potential side effects.

One of the great moments in the history of a new medicine is the report of its first clinical success. In the case of an antibiotic, the route is painstakingly long from the first culture to the first report of clinical response. But even then, a new drug has not yet been born. Development and production specialists must learn to produce and formulate it economically. Added long-term toxicological studies must be done. Tests must continue in a large number of new patients to determine the drug's value as a therapeutic agent and to document side effects. After these tests are completed, the sponsor submits a new drug application (NDA) to the Food and Drug Administration documenting safety and efficacy. Only after the FDA approves the NDA and its detailed labeling does the new product become available for prescribing by physicians.

Chemical Modification To Yield New Antibiotics

Back in the laboratory, microbiologists and chemists are already looking at another new antibiotic. Organic chemists are searching, too, with the same goal but a different approach. In the quest for better compounds to control specific diseases, they systematically modify structures of existing antibiotics by subjecting them to organic chemical reactions. Such changes in structure may enhance or extend antibacterial activity or may improve some accessory properties of the molecule.

For example, such a modification could improve the compound's ability to be absorbed from the gastrointestinal tract. If the acid stability of the molecule is increased, there may be a better chance it will survive transit through the stomach, thereby enhancing its usefulness in oral form. Such work is not without its frustrations. Many an organic chemist has declared that he has found a hundred ways to lose activity and not one way to improve it. Nevertheless, encouraged by successes seen in the modification of the tetracyclines, the penicillins and the cephalosporins, they continue experimenting.

Some years ago, a scientific report described the isolation of chlortetracycline from *Streptomyces aureofaciens.* Soon afterward, reports delineated the isolation of oxytetracycline from *Streptomyces rimosus.* Both of these compounds are active against a wide variety of pathogenic species and hence are called broad spectrum antibiotics. In these cases, two biologically active variants of the same basic structure were found in nature.

After they determined the complete structures of these antibiotics the chemists further varied the tetracycline structure in hopes of improving on some clinically important quality of the molecule. These efforts have been successful. (See Figure 3.)

Tetracycline, produced by catalytic removal of the chlorine from chlortetracycline, has proven superior to its parent compound. Complex chemical modification of oxytetracycline has yielded methacycline, and further variation of this compound, in turn, has produced doxycycline. Methacycline and doxycycline retain the antibacterial activity of the tetracycline group but possess enhanced lipid (or fat) solubility, providing for improved absorption and retention in the body. From superficial examination, the differences in chemical structure seem simple and uncomplicated, but the underlying chemistry is complex and difficult.

Biosynthesis of the Penicillins

The first member of the penicillin series was penicillin G. (See Figure 4.) During fermentation studies, chemists noted that by adding phenylacetic acid to the medium they could increase the yields. Phenylacetic acid is incorporated into the molecule during biosynthesis of the antibiotic. The organic acid acts as a precursor for the penicillin side chain. If compounds similar to phenylacetic acid are added to the fermentation medium, analogous penicillins can be produced. For example, phenoxyacetic acid is incorporated by the mold to yield penicillin V. Penicillin V is more stable in the stomach acids and can be taken orally, while penicillin G generally is given parenterally.

A number of penicillins have been made by such biosynthetic procedures. However, only organic acids that can be metabolized by the mold are potential penicillin precursors.

A turning point in penicillin chemistry occurred when the penicillin nucleus (6-aminopenicillanic acid or 6-APA) was discovered and characterized in penicillin fermentations. (See Figure 5.)

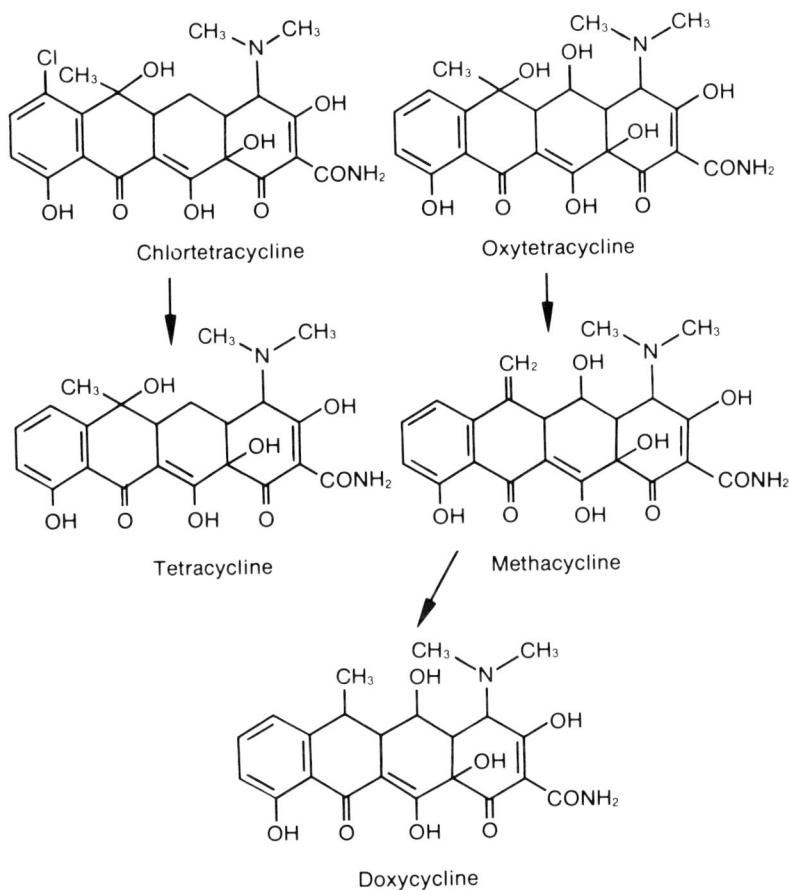

Figure 3. The natural tetracyclines chlortetracycline and oxytetracycline have been chemically modified to yield three clinically important derivatives: tetracycline, methacycline, and doxycycline.

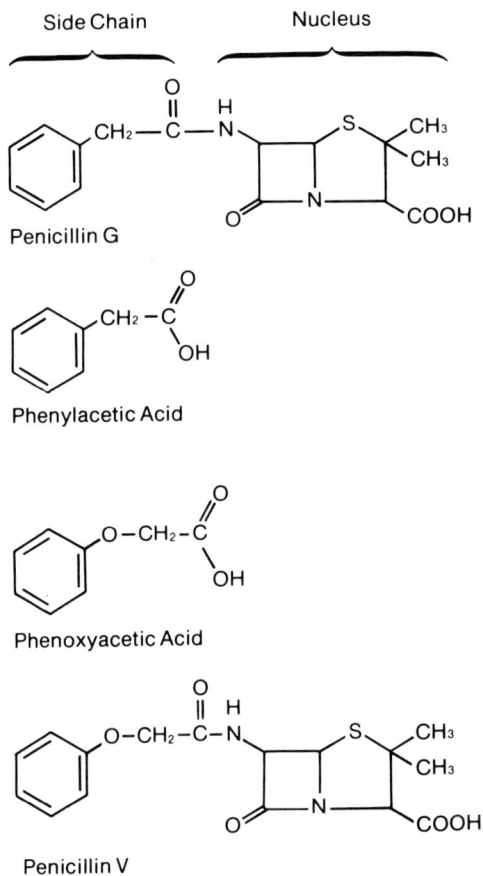

Figure 4. Phenylacetic acid is used by the *Penicillium* mold to produce penicillin G. Similarly, phenoxyacetic acid is used to produce penicillin V.

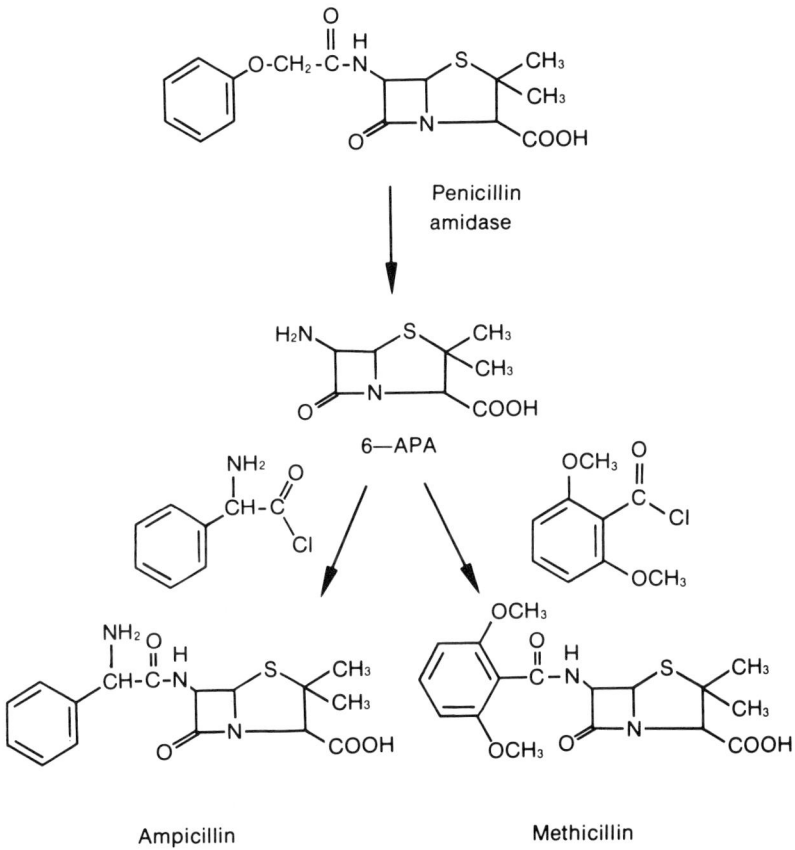

Figure 5. Penicillin V Is hydrolysed by the enzyme penicillin amidase yielding the penicillin nucleus, 6-amino-penicillanic acid. Acylation with the appropriate reagents yields ampicillin or methicillin.

If 6-APA could be supplied, a great number of new side chains could be attached to it chemically, without regard for the metabolic ability of the mold to handle the side chain. The potential for creating important new pencillins appeared to be immense. It was soon discovered that penicillin G or V can be hydrolyzed using a microbial enzyme, penicillin amidase, while 6-APA may be recovered in large amounts. Later, by application of acylation reactions, many new side chains were attached to the 6-APA.

Hundreds of new penicillins emerged from chemical laboratories, including two classes of clinically important compounds. The first is represented by ampicillin, which has a broader spectrum than penicillin G or V; that is, it has enhanced activity against gram-negative pathogens.

The second class of compounds is represented by methicillin and oxacillin. The chemical nature of the side chain confers on these compounds relative stability to penicillinase. Thus they can be used to treat penicillin-resistant infections.

A new antibiotic, cephalosporin C, has some structural similarities to the penicillins but is relatively stable to penicillinase. (See Figure 6.)

Plans were made to prepare the cephalosporin nucleus (7-ACA) and make new cephalosporins, via the acylation reaction, analogous to the preparation of penicillins. However, no amidase could be found to hydrolyze cephalosporin to yield 7-ACA. Therefore, the chemist had to devise a chemical reaction to accomplish hydrolysis. This was a formidable task, since the cephalosporin nucleus tended to disintegrate rather than separate from the side chain. In time, skill and ingenuity overcame the difficulties, and 7-ACA was produced. The acylation reactions were run, and a series of highly active compounds, including cephalothin, were prepared. Cephalothin is relatively stable to penicillinase and has unexpected and highly desirable activity against many gram-negative pathogens.

Thus, chemical modification has been an extremely useful technique for creating new and clinically useful medicines. Of course, these compounds must undergo the same rigorous proof

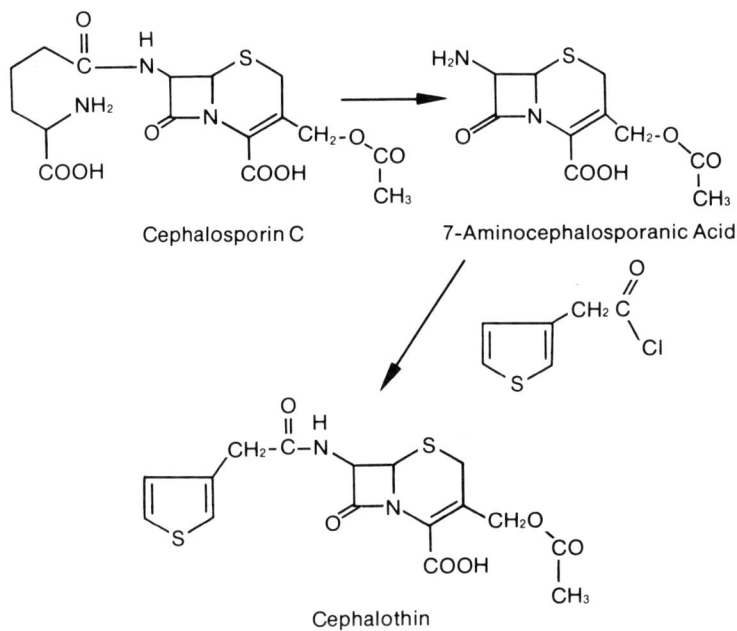

Figure 6. Cephalosporin C is cleaved chemically to yield the cephalosporin nucleus, 7-aminocephalosporanic acid. Acylation with thiophene-2-acetyl chloride yields cephalothin.

for safety and efficacy as the parent antibiotics before they become marketable products.

Conclusion

Today, Alexander Fleming's scientific heirs are probing into the microbial population of the world for other useful new antibiotics, and chemists are at work trying to improve the qualities of natural antibiotics. The search will go on, for infectious diseases—despite dramatic gains—still threaten the life and health of every human being. Tomorrow's search may well lead to the unexpected solution of the problem, but that is another story belonging to some future day.

Suggested Reading

Baldry, P. E. *The Battle Against Bacteria.* Cambridge: University Press, 1965.

Stewart, G. T. *The Penicillin Group of Drugs.* New York: Elsevier Publishing, 1965.

David, B. D., Dulbecco, R., Eisen, H. N., Ginsberg, H. S. & Wood, W. B. *Microbiology.* New York: Hoeber Medical Divison, Harper and Row, 1967.

Hahn, Peter. *Chemicals from Fermentation.* New York: Doubleday, 1968.

Garrod, L. P., & O'Grady, F. *Antibiotic and Chemotherapy.* (3rd. ed.) Edinburgh: Livingstone, 1971.

Flynn, E. H. *Cephalosporins and Penicillins—Chemistry and Biology.* New York: Academic Press, 1972.

CHAPTER 3

The Control of Pain

Frank H. Clarke
Naokata Yokoyama

Pain is the most important symptom of injury and disease, and mankind always has sought avidly for medicines to conquer pain. Drugs that relieve pain without causing loss of consciousness are known as analgesics.

Potent Analgesics

Before the dawn of organic chemistry in the late 19th century, most drugs were derived from plants. Opium, for example, is condensed sap from the unripe seed and capsule of the opium poppy. Use of opium dates from antiquity, and in 1680 the famous English physician Thomas Syndenham wrote, ". . . among remedies it has pleased Almighty God to give to man to relieve his sufferings, none is so universal and so efficacious as opium."

It was not until 1805, however, that morphine was isolated from opium by the German pharmacist, F. W. A. Serturner. Even then the age of potent analgesics had to await invention of the modern hypodermic syringe in 1850, because morphine is not as effective taken orally as it is given by injection. With the new technique, use of morphine to alleviate severe pain soon gained wide acceptance; it was commonly used to treat soldiers wounded in the American Civil War. The new pain remedy had its drawbacks, however, and problems of addiction in this country eventually became a serious liability.

It had long been known that habitual smoking or eating of opium caused physical dependence, and the ready availability of opium led to overuse. Still, the problem of addiction as a social

evil did not become pervasive until the advent of the hypodermic needle.

The important problem with the medical use of morphine
today is not so much its psychological effects as the tolerance
that develops in its prolonged use for treatment of chronic pain.
Progressively larger doses are needed to maintain the same degree of pain relief. As the doses become larger, side effects, such
as severe respiratory depression, finally limit the dose that can
be given safely. If morphine is then withdrawn to restore normal respiration, the patient suffers severe mental and physical
distress. This dual effect has often been called addiction liability, but scientists now prefer to call it mental and physical
dependence capacity. Such a serious detriment led to a search—
still going on—for a potent analgesic that does not cause physical dependence.

In early studies scientists chemically converted morphine to
its diacetyl derivative. The product, heroin, is more potent than
morphine and causes rapid and profound physiological effects,
including euphoria or a sense of well-being. Its continued use
leads to dependence, and illicit traffic in heroin rapidly became
a prominent social evil. Today, analgesics with a marked capacity to cause physical dependence, such as morphine and heroin,
are classed as narcotics and thus are subject to strict government
control. Heroin has such a strong physical dependence capacity
that it no longer has a legal use in therapy.

Mild and Moderate Analgesics

Some of the mild analgesics for the relief of less severe pain
also were derived from natural sources.

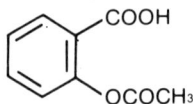

Aspirin

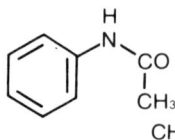

Acetanilid

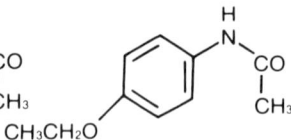

Acetophenetidin

Aspirin (acetylsalicylic acid) was first prepared in 1859. Its use in medicine began 40 years later following the discovery that salicylic acid is the active principle of the essential oil of Spirea ulmaria—an extract that had been in use for nearly a century to relieve pain and reduce fever. Salicyl alcohol, a closely related compound, is a component of the willow bark principle salicin, which was known to the ancients. Today aspirin is the most widely used medication for treating mild pain.

During the same era, another drama unfolded in the development of synthetic medicines. In 1886, when a pharmacist mistakenly filled a prescription for naphthalene (to treat intestinal parasites) with acetanilide, it was discovered that the patient's fever was reduced. Acetanilide soon became popular as an antipyretic (an agent that reduces fever) and as an analgesic. Later, when dangerous side effects of acetanilide were recognized, analogs and derivatives were prepared. One of these, acetophenetidine, turned out to be highly active and less toxic. Now widely used, it often is combined with aspirin for treating headache and pain caused by diseases involving muscles and joints.

Codeine, which effectively manages moderate pain, is the methyl ether of morphine, and it occurs naturally in opium in small amounts. It was prepared from morphine for the first time in 1881 and today finds extensive use in medicine, often as an antitussive agent to control coughing. Although it is classed as a narcotic, codeine is much weaker than morphine in its analgesic potency and its physical dependence capacity.

Morphine has a complex, three-dimensional structure (see appendix) which challenged organic chemists for more than a century. It was not until 1925, after hundreds of scientific papers had been written on the chemistry of morphine, that the correct structure was finally proposed by J. M. Gulland and Sir Robert Robinson.

Twenty-seven more years elapsed before scientists confirmed the accuracy of this structure. In 1952, Marshall Gates announced the total synthesis of morphine, and Gilbert Stork described its stereochemistry (spatial arrangement of atoms in the molecule).

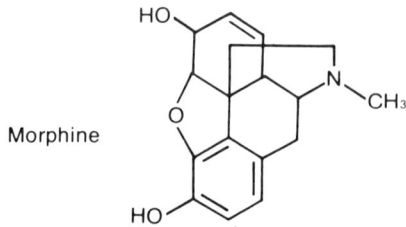

Morphine

Gulland and Robinson (1925)

In the picture opposite, a space-filling model of morphine has beside it a skeletal model to show more clearly the relative orientation of each of the atoms. The structural formula can be drawn so that it represents the stereochemical configuration as depicted in the skeletal model. It can be seen that a basic tertiary nitrogen atom is contained in a piperidine ring, the plane of which is perpendicular to the plane of the aromatic ring. With such a complex structure it is small wonder that modification of morphine presented enormous problems for the synthetic chemist; he was attempting to develop a more potent analgesic without a sure knowledge of what he was trying to modify.

Nevertheless, in 1929, a team directed by Dr. Lyndon Small, a chemist, and Dr. Nathan Eddy, a pharmacologist, set out to prepare a morphine derivative with improved properties. They worked under the auspices of the newly formed Committee on Drug Addiction of the National Research Council. Their work was stimulated by the knowledge that small changes in the morphine structure, for example, in codeine and heroin, created profound changes in physiological properties. They prepared about 120 morphine derivatives and evaluated them pharmacologically. They found no analgesically active morphine derivative without physical dependence capacity. During this period the stage was set for future discoveries. Many of these developments were reported to the Committee on Drug Addiction (now the Committee on Problems of Drug Dependence) which meets annually to discuss the results of analgesic research in laboratories all over the world. Today the Committee also supports research and provides facilities for pharmacological and clinical evaluation of new analgesics for physical dependence capacity.

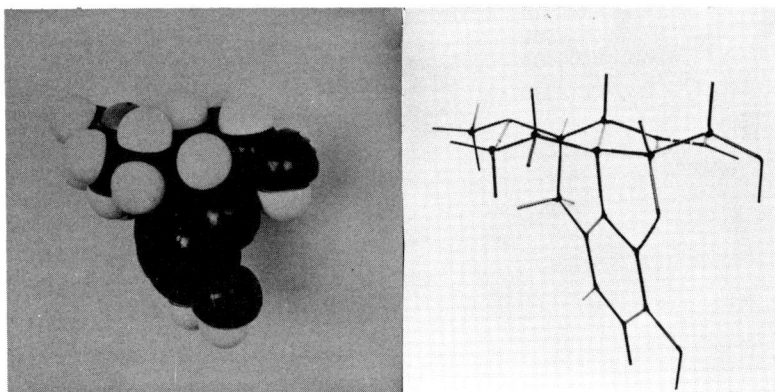

Figure 1. The space filling Corey-Pauling-Koltun model of morphine shown on the left should be compared with the skeletal model of morphine on the right built with Dreiding stereomodels.

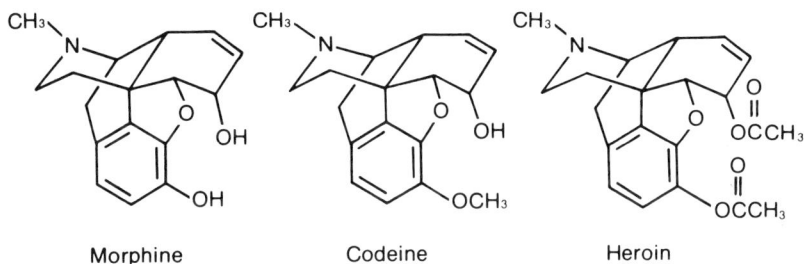

Morphine   Codeine   Heroin

The Heritage of Atropine

In 1939, modifications of naturally occurring drugs again played a decisive role in the development of analgesics. In that year the chemist O. Eisleb and the pharmacologist O. Schaumann, reported on their work at I. G. Farbenindustrie with a relatively simple phenylpiperidine ester which was intended to have improved properties as an antispasmodic. The structure of the new ester partly corresponded with that of atropine, a naturally occurring antispasmodic. However, tests proved the new piperidine ester was a potent analgesic. Currently, next to opiates, this ester (commonly known as meperidine) is probably the most widely used narcotic analgesic. At first the relation of meperidine to morphine went unrecognized; its effects were believed to be quite different.

Today, after years of clinical experience, scientists have demonstrated that meperidine also causes physical dependence—although not to the same degree as morphine.

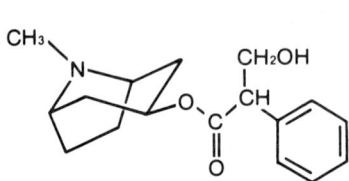

Atropine

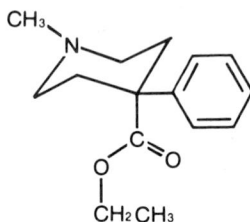

Meperidine

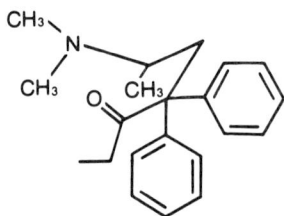

Methadone

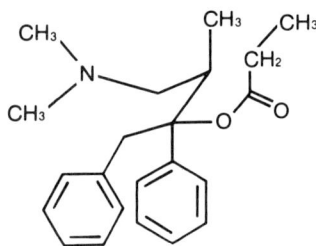

Propoxyphene

The discovery of meperidine encouraged further research at I. G. Farbenindustrie. Carried out in Germany during World War II, this work led to still another potent analgesic known in the U.S. as methadone. Methadone has most of the side effects of morphine but has the advantage of oral effectiveness. It also causes physical dependence, but the symptoms produced on abrupt withdrawal are much milder than those of morphine. In fact, the most important use of methadone today is in treatment of heroin addicts.

A wide variety of modifications of methadone were synthesized as U.S. research continued. One of these, d-propoxyphene, was prepared in 1955 by Albert Pohland of the Lilly Laboratories. d-Propoxyphene lacks the high potency of morphine and is not subject to the strict controls of narcotic analgesics. It is now widely used in combination with aspirin.

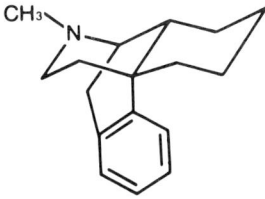

N-Methylmorphinan

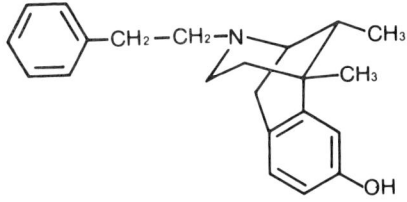

Phenazocine

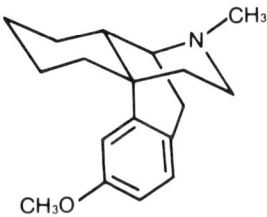

Dextromethorphan

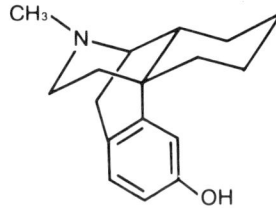

Levorphanol

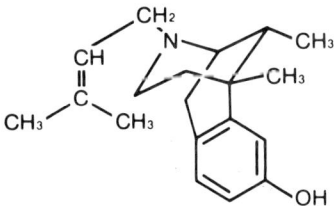

Pentazocine

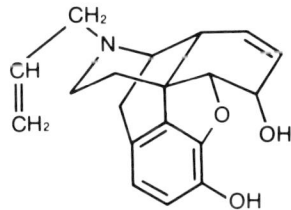

Nalorphine

Morphine Simplification

In 1925, Sir Robert Robinson and his co-workers suggested a possible way by which morphine could be biosynthesized from simpler compounds in the poppy plant. These biogenetic hypotheses were applied in principle by Rudolf Grewe to the first synthesis of a compound with the complete tetracyclic carbon-nitrogen skeleton of morphine. The product, N-methylmorphinan, has 20 percent of the analgesic activity of morphine.

Later O. Schnider and A. Grüssner, and also Grewe and his associates synthesized an N-methylmorphinan derivative with a phenolic hydroxyl group in the appropriate position. This compound was resolved into its optical isomers and the levorotatory isomer became known as levorphanol, a clinically useful analgesic effective when taken orally. Unfortunately, it also causes physical dependence and is thereby subject to narcotic controls. On the other hand, the dextrorotatory isomer was converted to its O-methyl ether and has become a useful product known as dextromethorphan. It is devoid of analgesic activity and is free of physical dependence capacity. It is widely used as an orally effective antitussive.

Everette May and his associates carried still further the simplification of the morphine structure. Beginning in 1954, they prepared many tricyclic compounds called benzomorphans. Some of them were effective analgesics with a greatly reduced physical dependence capacity, and one compound, phenazocine, is clinically useful. Phenazocine is more potent than morphine; however it has a physical dependence liability and is still classed as a narcotic.

Meanwhile, another achievement, the discovery of pentazocine, a benzomorphan derivative, opened a unique new pathway.

The Antagonist Story

In 1943 Klause Unna demonstrated that a morphine derivative, nalorphine (a compound in which the methyl group is replaced by an allyl substituent) antagonized or cancelled most of the pharmacological effects of morphine. This led Louis Lasagna and Henry Beecher, in 1954, to test the combination of morphine and nalorphine in man. Nalorphine itself had not been shown to be analgesic in animals, but they hoped that—as an antagonist—it would reverse the undesirable features of morphine without destroying the analgesia. They used nalorphine itself in a control experiment, and the compound soon exhibited undesirable psychotomimetic effects, which rendered it impractical as a drug either alone or in combination. Most disturbing of these effects were hallucinations and disorientation.

However, in these experiments researchers discovered that nalorphine as an analgesic in man has a potency equal to morphine. Other researchers, Arthur Keats and Jane Telford, soon confirmed this finding. Furthermore, it was known that nalorphine, with its antagonist properties, would not support morphine addiction. On the contrary, when administered to a morphine addict it immediately precipitated typical morphine withdrawal symptoms.

Taking advantage of these properties of nalorphine, Sydney Archer and his associates, and also Maxwell Gordon and his co-workers, synthesized a series of derivatives of the benzomorphan class of analgesics with allyl substituents on the nitrogen atom. After studies in animals, several were selected for extensive clinical trials. One of them was pentazocine. Although not as potent as morphine when taken orally, pentazocine does have the advantage of not being classified as causing morphine-like physical dependence in man. Since a potent oral analgesic with ideal properties has not yet been found, the search continues today with more intensity than ever. Meanwhile, the possibility of using morphine antagonists for the treatment of narcotic addiction is also receiving more attention.

The Search for a Rational Approach

We have briefly traced various pathways in the development of safe and effective analgesics. The story began in the latter part of the 19th century with a search for analogs of pain-relieving drugs of natural origin that would be free from undesirable side effects. These diverse pathways seem to be leading in different directions. At first glance, the structure of propoxyphene appears to have little in common with that of morphine or of the benzomorphans. Yet, as illustrated above, there may be a relationship. The most active of these analgesics all seem to have some features in common: an aromatic ring *a*, a quaternary carbon atom *b* to which ring *a* is attached and a tertiary nitrogen atom separated from the quaternary carbon by a chain *c* of two carbon atoms.

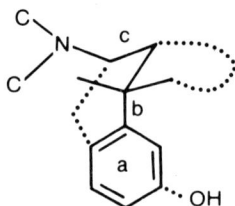

Structural Features of Analgesics

Several authors have postulated that there must be a receptor with a specific affinity for active analgesic molecules. This classical hypothesis of the drug-receptor interaction has evolved from a fascinating study of structure-activity relationships. Although this hypothesis is helpful to the medicinal chemist in the design of new analgesics, it is by no means as valuable as an understanding of what the nature of the receptor site might be.

In their pharmacological and biochemical aspects, some other areas of medicinal research have had parallel development. For instance, theories of hypotensive drugs' receptor sites and of the mechanism of their action have emerged during development stages. Such theories have helped in designing improved medicines for lowering blood pressure. In other areas, too, we are beginning to understand the nature of drug action. Unfortunately, there is still no receptor site theory of analgesia that is universally accepted.

We are only beginning to understand the phenomenon of pain. In animals we usually measure pain through reflex actions—twitching of a tail, lifting of a paw, or a vocal response—elicited by noxious stimuli such as heat. These tests can indicate that an analgesic might slow the reflex response, for example, of abruptly removing a burned finger when we touch a hot stove inadvertently. But what about their practical consequences? Will the test compound be as effective for the deep pain of intestinal cancer as it is in blocking the reflex response? The patient may know the cancer has not disappeared, and the dulling of his senses does not necessarily alleviate fear that accompanies his pain.

The most potent analgesics apparently act centrally in the brain where the pain as such is perceived. What is the mechanism of the central effect that results in a sensation of pain? Some recent biochemical and pharmacological experiments relate this phenomenon to one or another of such natural hormones as serotonin or acetylcholine. These studies and their implications are far from clear. There have been a number of hypotheses, but no one has yet identified the nature of the analgesic receptor. Problems such as these remain a stern challenge to the medicinal chemist and to his collaborators in the biological and biochemical sciences. Hopefully, as the solution unfolds, new and better medicines will be designed, and the safe relief of intolerable pain will one day be achieved.

Suggested Reading

Archer, S. (et al.) *Narcotic Antagonists as Analgesics*, Laboratory Aspects; pp. 162–169; Keats, A. S., & Telford, J., *Narcotic Antagonists as Analgesics*, Clinical Aspects, pp. 170–176. In *Molecular Modification in Drug Design*, Advances in Chemistry Series, 45. Washington, D.C.: American Chemical Society, 1964.

Archer, S., & Harris, L. S. *Narcotic Antagonists—Progress in Drug Research*. Vol. 8. Basel: Birkhauser Verlag, 1965.

deStevens, G. (Ed.) *Analgetics*. Vol. 5. *Medicinal Chemistry*. New York: Academic Press, 1965.

Eddy, N. B., & May, D. L. Synthetic Analgesics. Part IIB. *Benzomorphans*. New York: Pergamon Press, 1966.

Hallerbach, J. (et al.) Synthetic Analgesics. Part IIA. *Morphinans*. New York: Pergamon Press, 1966.

Holmes, H. L., & Stork, G. *The Alkaloids*. Vol. 2. *The Morphine Alkaloids*. New York: Academic Press, 1952.

Janssen, P. A. J. Synthetic Analgesics. Part I. *Diphenylpropyl-amines*. New York: Pergamon Press, 1960.

Library of Davidson College

Mellett, L. B., & Woods, L. A. *Analgesia and Addiction.* Vol. 5. *Progress in Drug Research.* Basel: Birkhauser Verlag, 1963.

Small, L. F., & Lutz, R. E. *Chemistry of the Opium Alkaloids,* (U.S. Public Health Reports: Supplement No. 103 to the Public Health Report) Washington, D.C.: United States Government Printing Office, 1932.

CHAPTER 4

The Sulfa Drugs and Their Legacy

W. M. McLamore

The story of sulfa drugs and their remarkable legacy properly begins with Paul Ehrlich (1854–1915). Physician, bacteriologist and immunologist, Ehrlich made uncommon use of the rapidly developing chemical knowledge of his time. He was the first to adopt the multidisciplinary approach so characteristic of modern drug research. Several of the concepts that he first formulated remain central to the thinking of present-day medicinal chemists.

The major killers of the 19th century were the infectious diseases, and Ehrlich sought with great drive and imagination to find "magic bullets" against the responsible microorganisms. He coined the still useful term *chemotherapy* to describe the destruction of these minute invaders by chemical agents that would not be too damaging to the tissues of the human or animal host. Ehrlich found such an agent against the tiny parasite (spirochete) that causes syphilis, but the chemotherapy of bacterial diseases remained an elusive goal for some years after his death. The conquest of these common and costly diseases—so far advanced in this age of antibiotics—began, curiously enough, with the dyestuff industry.

Nineteenth century bacteriologists initiated the staining of bacteria with dyes in their efforts to make these tiny organisms more visible under the microscope. Such stains are still widely used today, and an important classification system for bacteria (Gram-positive, Gram-negative) is based on the staining technique devised by Christian Gram. Paul Ehrlich was well aware of the implications of dye staining to the search for antibacterial drugs, and he contributed substantially to this field. It was not

41

difficult to find dyes lethal to bacteria, but some of these same dyes also stained and damaged animal cells. Hence the problem: Find a dye sufficiently selective for bacterial cells. The biochemistry of all living cells is similar in so many ways that it is not surprising to find this problem of selectivity of drug action still very much with us today.

From Dye Chemistry to Drug Therapy

The first sign that such selectivity had been achieved came in 1935, with the discovery that the deep red dye sulfamidochrysoidine (Prontosil) protected mice against severe and normally fatal streptococcal infections. This advance by G. Domagk and his co-workers, in the German laboratories of I. G. Farbenindustrie, ushered in the modern era of antibacterial chemotherapy. For his breakthrough, G. Domagk received a Nobel Prize in 1938. Like most discoveries, this one had a long history, and from our vantage point it is hard to see why such an accomplishment had not taken place earlier.

Sulfamidochrysoidine belongs to the important class of azo dyes, and contains the sulfonamide group (circled in the formulas below). Such dyes had been known for some years to bind more tightly to the animal fibers silk and wool and were prized for their color fastness in laundering. It was also widely known, even in Ehrlich's time, that bacteria were similar to wool in their binding of dyes. Most surprisingly, as early as 1917, W. A. Jacobs and M. Heidelberger had shown that other sulfonamide-containing azo dyes had antibacterial activity. But no one followed up their discoveries.

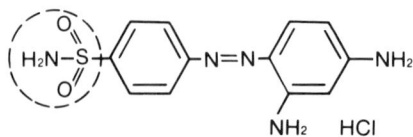

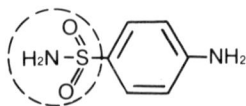

Prontosil   Sulfanilamide

One puzzling point about sulfamidochrysoidine, however, was its much greater antibacterial activity in the living animal (*in vivo*) than in the test tube (*in vitro*); as we know even better today, the reverse is almost always true. It seemed as though the animal must be changing the drug in some way to make it more effective. This proved to be the case; a French group at the Pasteur Institute soon discovered that the active drug, sulfanilamide, was a fragment of the sulfamidochrysoidine molecule, and no longer a dye. This finding was soon confirmed in other countries, and the modern era of antibacterial chemotherapy had truly been launched.

The Sulfa Drugs

Although sulfanilamide was a lifesaving drug in many severe human infections, it had several drawbacks, the most serious being the kidney damage that sometimes occurred with high doses. Medicinal chemists quickly rose to this challenge and ultimately produced almost 5,000 sulfa drugs—all of them derivatives of sulfanilamide. Two of the most successful have been sulfathiazole and sulfadiazine.

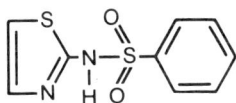

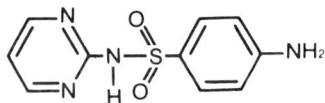

Sulfathiazole   Sulfadiazine

Although they have been less commonly prescribed since the advent of antibiotics, the sulfonamides (or sulfa drugs) still find considerable use in modern medicine.

The mode of action of the sulfonamide drugs sparked great interest. For one thing, sulfanilamide, unlike the older antiseptics, did not kill bacteria outright but simply arrested their normally rapid multiplication and thereby allowed the natural defenses of the body to finish the job. D. D. Woods and P. Fildes in 1940 independently showed that the antibacterial action of sulfanilamide could be overcome by providing the bacteria with large amounts of p-aminobenzoic acid, a natural substance required by many bacteria for normal growth and reproduction. The close structural resemblance of these two molecules is illustrated by their formulas.

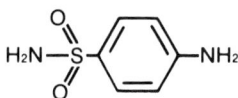

Sulfanilamide   p-Aminobenzoic Acid

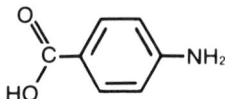

Metabolite Antagonism

This key observation not only suggested a possible mode of action for sulfanilamide, but brought to the fore the general concept of *metabolite antagonism,* which continues to play an important role in drug design to this day. Briefly, this concept calls for exposing a cell, bacterial or otherwise, whose growth and development it is desired to inhibit, to a relatively high concentration of a chemical compound (drug) that closely resembles a natural substance, or metabolite, required by the cell for normal growth and development. The unnatural compound cannot be utilized by the cell, but competes with the natural metabolite for uptake into the cell, or otherwise prevents its utilization by the cell. In short, the unnatural substance (drug) behaves as an antagonist to a natural, essential cell metabolite. Deliberate attempts to use this concept for drug discovery so far have met with only modest success, and notably in the field of cancer chemotherapy. Still, in its most general sense, metabolite antagonism is bound to become more useful as we learn intimate details of biochemical pathways that we would like to control.

Diuretics

The next stage of our story begins, like so many in drug discovery, with a chance clinical observation. Patients taking sulfanilamide often excreted a larger than usual volume of urine that was more alkaline than normal. Researchers soon discovered that sulfanilamide blocks (inhibits) the enzyme carbonic anhydrase which is found in many organs of the body, including the kidney, where its role is to acidify urine. There existed a real medical need at the time for better and safer diuretic drugs—medications to counteract the fluid retention of heart failure, kidney disease and other ailments by increasing the output of salts and water in the urine.

This was a situation made to order for the chemist-biochemist-pharmacologist medicinal team. Testing soon began on many sulfonamides, either as inhibitors (blockers) of the isolated enzyme, carbonic anhydrase, or as diuretic agents in animals. It shortly become apparent, particularly to a group at the Lederle Laboratories, headed by R. H. Roblin, that the best enzyme inhibitors—and diuretics—were found among the more acidic sulfonamides. This led them to make and test a series of still more acidic, heterocyclic sulfonamides. One of these, acetazolamide, reached the market as the first of a new class of diuretic drugs.

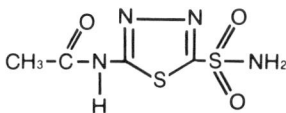

Acetazolamide   Carzenide

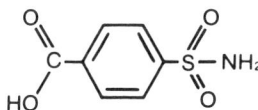

Acetazolamide has been largely superseded by more effective diuretics, but the research that culminated in its discovery still ranks as one of the best examples of the correlation of a physical property (acidity) of the drug molecule with its biological activity. As such, it has strongly influenced the thinking of all medicinal chemists in their perpetual search for more rational approaches to drug design. Moreover, among many other diuretics inspired by acetazolamide, several of which eventually reached the market, the experimental drug carzenide was of special interest. This agent, though it was never marketed, proved to be the key to the future of diuretic research, as we shall see a bit later.

Antidiabetic Drugs

Meanwhile, in the continuing quest for superior antibacterial drugs among the sulfonamides, another critical clinical observation occurred. Patients in France under treatment for typhoid fever with a new, experimental sulfa drug, IPTD (an abbreviation of the chemical name), showed all the symptoms of low blood sugar. This observation of the blood-sugar lowering or

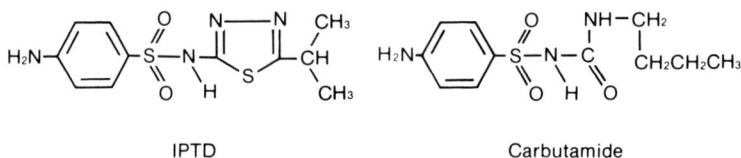

IPTD   Carbutamide

hypoglycemic action of IPTD, made in 1942 by M. Janbon and co-workers, was pursued thoroughly in animals by A. Loubatières during and after the war. But the long-standing hope for an orally effective and safe hypoglycemic drug, to replace the frequent insulin injections required by diabetics, remained a dream until some years later.

It was not until 1955 that H. Franke and J. Fuchs rediscovered this class of oral antidiabetic drugs. While studying in man the anti-infective properties of yet another experimental sulfonamide, carbutamide, they also observed symptoms of low blood sugar. This time, however, the practical therapeutic implications were not overlooked, and carbutamide soon was available to physicians in Europe for treatment of diabetes.

To the medicinal chemist, IPTD and carbutamide, however different they may look to the uninitiated, are clearly sisters under the skin. Carbutamide, though, proved to be the more useful lead in the intensive work on related compounds that now occupied many laboratories. Carbutamide is a *sulfonylurea,* and this generic term also fits those of its descendants that have reached the marketplace—at least until very recently. Sulfonylurea drugs cannot replace insulin for those severe diabetics who develop the disease early in life. But they have revolutionized treatment for the much more numerous diabetics who are not afflicted until their middle years. The sulfonylureas act by releasing insulin from the pancreas, and maturity-onset diabetics, unlike the early or juvenile type, still have some insulin-producing capacity in their pancreatic cells.

The initial break for the medicinal chemist was the finding, in the German laboratories of Farbwerke Hoechst, that the amino group of carbutamide (and IPTD), while essential for antibacterial properties, is not essential for its hypoglycemic action. The first drug that resulted from this finding, tolbutamide, also became the first sulfonylurea made available to patients in the U.S. Like all subsequent sulfonylureas, tolbutamide is devoid of antibacterial properties, which is perhaps an advantage in treating diabetes.

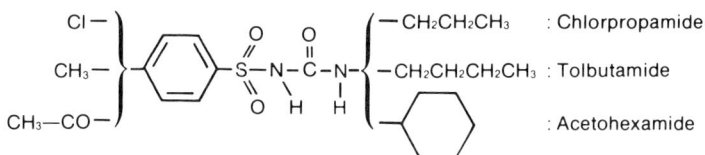

The structural diagram shows substituents $Cl-$, CH_3-, CH_3-CO- on a benzene ring connected to $-S(=O)(=O)-N(O)-C(=O)-N(H)(H)-$ group, with terminal groups $-CH_2CH_2CH_3$: Chlorpropamide, $-CH_2CH_2CH_2CH_3$: Tolbutamide, and a cyclohexyl ring : Acetohexamide.

Tolbutamide has, however, brief duration of action, owing to the rapid oxidation in man of the p-methyl group, to give a metabolite which is inactive. (The word *metabolite* is used in a somewhat different sense here than earlier in the chapter.) This characteristic, and the resultant need for frequent administration, was overcome in chlorpropamide, the second sulfonylurea drug to become available in the U.S. Since the p-chloro group of chlorpropamide cannot be oxidized and the drug is excreted by the kidney very slowly, it need be given only once a day and in lower doses. The more recently introduced drug acetohexamide has an intermediate duration of action. Hence physicians have a range of choices for oral treatment of maturity-onset diabetics.

Probenecid and Kidney Function

Before resuming our account of modern diuretic research, we should mention a related drug containing the sulfonamide group, namely probenecid. Not only is probenecid of considerable therapeutic importance in its own right but, like the sulfonamide diuretics, it has contributed to our knowledge of the kidney and how it functions. Moreover, probenecid resulted from an unusually rational and well-planned approach to a specific therapeutic objective.

Despite heroic efforts by the U.S. drug industry, penicillin remained in short supply during World War II and for some time

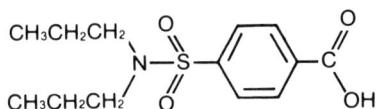

Probenecid

thereafter. One reason was the massive doses required to treat the more severe infections, because penicillin is rapidly eliminated from the body by way of the kidneys. Penicillin is an organic acid, and a special transport system in the kidney speeds the elimination of such acids. Dr. Karl Beyer and his associates at the Sharp and Dohme research laboratories observed that it should be possible to find a simple organic acid, not otherwise harmful, that would compete with penicillin for this special transport system and thereby slow down its excretion through the kidneys. They chose the sulfonamide drugs as the logical beginning for their examination, since as a class they are unusually well tolerated and already were known to act on the kidney (cf. acetazolamide). In the ensuing search, which must then have been relatively uncomplicated from the technical point of view, probenecid emerged as an agent with all the desired properties.

As penicillin production increased, use of probenecid for its penicillin-sparing action became less important. Meanwhile another valuable medical action of the drug had been unveiled, and probenecid is widely used today to treat chronic gout. In this ancient affliction of mankind, pain arises from deposition of uric acid in the joints of the body. Uric acid is a natural end-product of body metabolism, but to the kidney it is just another organic acid. In this case, probenecid competes with uric acid for a transport system that leads to reabsorption of uric acid in the kidney. The net result is an increase in the urinary excretion of uric acid and a decrease in the abnormally high body levels of this acid that characterize chronic gout.

Probenecid is closely related structurally to the diuretic agent carzenide, mentioned above. Probenecid, in fact, must have been derived from carzenide by replacement of the two hydrogen atoms on the sulfonamide nitrogen with other groups. Such derivatives of the sulfonamide diuretics had been known from earlier research to be devoid of diuretic activity, unless the replacement groups could be removed readily by the body. The propyl groups in probenecid are not so removed, and the drug works precisely because its actions on the kidney exclude the diuretic action of its parent compound.

As noted earlier, carzenide proved to be the key to future diuretic research. Like acetazolamide and other sulfonamide diuretics that act by inhibiting the enzyme carbonic anhydrase, carzenide also revealed its built-in Achilles heel. All these drugs caused an alkaline urine, in effect increasing the excretion of sodium bicarbonate. This resulted ultimately in metabolic acidosis—an electrolyte (ionic) imbalance of the body—which was not only undesirable in itself but completely prevented any further diuretic action by the drug. The ideal diuretic, on the other hand, would simply increase the volume of urine without changing its composition. To do this, it would have to promote excretion of equal amounts of sodium and chloride ions— sodium chloride (or common salt) being a major constituent of normal urine. This essentially is what the earlier mercurial diuretics did, and they were the most effective diuretics known at the time; unfortunately, they had to be given by injection and also presented serious toxicity problems.

Sulfonamides Yield New Diuretics

Most research groups that had been working on sulfonamide diuretics must have become discouraged by the fact that the major limitations of these drugs seemed to be intrinsic to their mode of action. But the Sharp and Dohme group astutely noted

that carzenide, although primarily a carbonic anhydrase inhibitor, nevertheless produced a slight increase in chloride (or
sodium chloride) excretion, both in dogs and in man. In the
best scientific tradition, the significance of this observation,
unimpressive in itself, was not lost on prepared minds. Systematic pursuit of this finding by a team of pharmacologists and
medicinal chemists, headed by Dr. Karl Beyer and Dr. James
Sprague, respectively, led to one of the great successes of modern medicine.

The first break in studying the effect of various sulfonamide
derivatives on chloride excretion came with the compound
dichlorphenamide. Introduction of a second sulfonamide group,
in a specific position relative to the first, considerably enhanced
chloride excretion, even though the compound was still a potent carbonic anhydrase inhibitor. Dichlorphenamide had
enough advantages over earlier diuretics to reach the market,
but it is used today chiefly in glaucoma, an eye disorder amena-
ble to treatment with carbonic anhydrase inhibitors. The ideal
diuretic was not yet in hand.

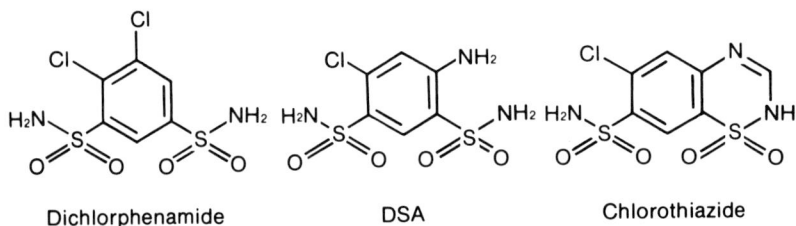

Dichlorphenamide　　　　　DSA　　　　　Chlorothiazide

The big break came for this group of scientists (by now part
of the Merck, Sharp and Dohme organization) while they were
studying the reactions of a close analog of dichlorphenamide.
This analog, which was given the abbreviated name *DSA*, can
also be regarded as a derivative of the familiar sulfanilamide,
with the addition of the second sulfonamide group and one of
the chloro groups of dichlorphenamide. The diuretic actions of
DSA itself were of interest, but far more intriguing was the
novel heterocyclic derivative chlorothiazide, produced by the
action of formic acid on DSA. Chlorothiazide proved to be a

potent diuretic in animals and in man. Although it retained moderate activity as an inhibitor of carbonic anhydrase, it led to marked chloride excretion as well. Here, then, was a nearly ideal diuretic, highly effective orally and producing a urine of almost normal ionic composition. The medical uses of chlorothiazide proved to be even broader than had been anticipated; it clearly represents one of the most striking therapeutic advances of recent years.

Varying the Thiazide Molecule

One drawback of chlorothiazide, however, is the rather large dose required for maximum clinical effect. From the efforts of other research groups that subsequently entered the field, it soon became apparent that structural variation of the thiazide molecule could lead to agents effective at much smaller doses. Ultimately, quite a few thiazide diuretics became available, all clearly inspired by chlorothiazide, some of them effective at a dose hundreds of times smaller than that of chlorothiazide. Apart from other possible advantages of these more potent thiazides, one reason for their acceptance surely is the reluctance of physicians to expose their patients to any larger amount of medicine than necessary.

Chlorothiazide and the other thiazides have been unusually successful medications, but they are not without defects. One of their most serious deficiencies is their limited effectiveness in severe cases of salt and fluid retention. Recent research has led to products that are even more effective in such conditions. Not surprisingly, one of these is a sulfonamide, furosemide.

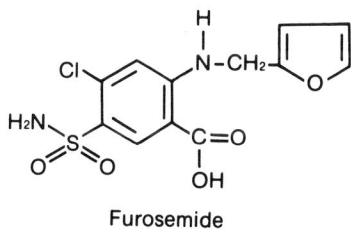

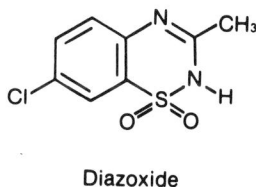

Furosemide   Diazoxide

The major medical use of the thiazides today is not as diuretics but as antihypertensive agents for reducing high blood pressure. In fact, the antihypertensive action of chlorothiazide was discovered quite early in clinical studies. Here, too, the effectiveness of the thiazides is somewhat limited, and severely hypertensive patients usually require other drugs as well. But the thiazides are so well tolerated that they are almost always the first to be tried, except in the most severe cases. Even in these instances, fortunately, thiazides potentiate the action of the more powerful medications, allowing them to be used in smaller, better tolerated doses.

Antihypertensive Agents

Depletion of body salt and water with low-salt diets had long been standard treatment for hypertension, so it was natural to suppose that the thiazides lower blood pressure as a result of their diuretic action. Evidence gradually accumulated, however, that there must be another, more direct antihypertensive action. This line of thought led to an interesting experimental drug from the Schering laboratories—diazoxide. As indicated by the structural formula above, diazoxide is a slightly modified version of the chlorothiazide nucleus but without the free sulfonamide group. In seeking to dissociate the diuretic and antihypertensive actions of chlorothiazide, this was a logical approach to take, since earlier work had shown that the free sulfonamide group is essential for satisfactory diuretic activity. Diazoxide proved to be a more potent antihypertensive agent than the thiazides; not only was it free of diuretic activity but, surprisingly, it had an antidiuretic action. The latter could be overcome by coadministration of a thiazide, but this combination produced a rather serious side effect; namely, an elevation in blood sugar (hyperglycemia). These unexpected findings with diazoxide have, in turn, stimulated research that promises, among other things, to help explain how insulin is released from its storage sites in the pancreas.

Diazoxide has been available in England for several years, not only for emergency treatment of hypertension but for use in those relatively rare conditions characterized by low blood sugar (hypoglycemia). Just recently, an intravenous form of the drug has been approved in the U.S. for emergency treatment of malignant hypertension.

Whatever its limitations as an antihypertensive agent for general (long term) use, diazoxide is an important research lead, because it lowers blood pressure by a mechanism that is widely considered to be ideal—a direct relaxant effect on the blood vessels. It seems likely, therefore, that diazoxide looms large in the thinking of the many research teams around the world who are seeking safer, more effective medications for lowering blood pressure. This strongly suggests that the legacy of the sulfa drugs, impressive as we have seen it to be, may be by no means exhausted.

Suggested Reading

Beyer, K. H., & Baer, J. E. Newer Diuretics. In E. Jucker (Ed.), *Progress in Drug Research.* Vol. 2. Basel: Birkhauser Verlag, 1960.

Burger, A. *Medicinal Chemistry.* (3rd ed.) New York, Wiley-Interscience, 1970.

Campbell, G. D. Oral Hypoglycemic Agents. Pharmacology and Therapeutics, *Medicinal Chemistry*, Vol. 9, New York, Academic Press, 1969.

deStevens, G. Diuretics—Chemistry and Pharmacology. *Medicinal Chemistry*, Vol. 1, New York: Academic Press, 1963.

Goodman, L. S., & Gilman, A. *The Pharmacological Basis of Therapeutics.* (4th ed.) New York: MacMillan, 1970.

Hawking, F., & Lawrence, J. S. *The Sulfonamides.* London: H. K. Lewis, 1950.

Loubatieres, A. The Use of Certain Sulfonamides in the Treatment of Experimental Diabetes Mellitus. *Annals of the New York Academy of Sciences*, 1956, 67 185-206.

CHAPTER 5

To Tranquilizers and Antidepressants From Antimalarials and Antihistamines

Charles L. Zirkle

Bedlam is a common name for the hospital of St. Mary of Bethlehem in Lambeth, London, first founded as a religious house but used as an asylum for the mentally ill as early as the 15th century. Until the middle of the 20th century, the word *bedlam* aptly connoted the prevailing conditions in most hospital wards where severely agitated mental patients (psychotics) were detained and, frequently, restrained.

Early in 1952, a 57-year-old laborer was admitted to a French mental institution because of his erratic, uncontrollable behavior. He had made impassioned political speeches in cafes, proclaimed love of liberty while walking down the streets with a flower pot and assaulted strangers. Doctors decided to try giving him a new drug, later named chlorpromazine. Within a day the patient was calmer, and a week later he was joking with the medical staff. After three weeks he appeared almost normal and was soon discharged. The doctors observed that other agitated, hyperactive patients also benefitted from the drug. Thus began a revolution in the therapy of mental illness—a revolution that brought forth not only chemical means of alleviating symptoms but also a change in attitudes toward these terrible diseases.

The enthusiasm over the discovery of chlorpromazine was mixed with skepticism—for good reason. Many methods of treating psychotic patients had been tried before with little success. The usual central nervous system (CNS) depressants, such as the sedatives, calmed only when given in large doses that usually made the patient stuporous. Psychoanalysis, frequently used as a treatment of neuroses (milder forms of mental illness), was not practical for the treatment of large numbers of hospital-

ized, psychotic patients. Some clinical advances were achieved
by use of insulin coma and electroshock therapy, introduced in
the 1930s. Numerous patients benefitted from these rather drastic and complicated treatments, but only highly trained medical
personnel can administer them safely. In many institutions the
number of beds required for psychiatric patients continued to
rise at a discouragingly rapid rate. Many mental hospitals still
looked more like houses of detention than places for rehabilita-
tion and cure.

Antipsychotic Agents

Then came chlorpromazine and related drugs to calm
hyperagitated psychiatric patients and alleviate symptoms of
their illnesses without clouding consciousness or causing other
incapacitating effects. Unlike some other CNS depressants, such
as morphine and the barbiturates, the new agents are
nonaddicting and do not produce psychological dependence.
The patients usually become more cooperative and take part in
occupational, recreational and psychotherapies. Benefits have
extended far beyond those accorded the individual patient.
Within mental hospitals an attitude of hopefulness and con-
fidence toward the psychoses has replaced one of pessimism and
despair. Hospitalized patients can be actively treated, not merely detained. An impressive decrease in numbers of patients and
in average length of hospitalization has taken place. In addition,
with the help of the new medications many patients can be
cared for in their communities without hospitalization.

Figure   1   dramatically   illustrates   the   impact   of
chlorpromazine and other psychopharmacological agents on
mental hospital populations. They largely brought about the
steady decline in the number of patients in government mental
hospitals beginning in 1955. Instead of an estimated increase of
120–150 thousand patients between 1955 and 1967 based on
the rate of admissions before 1955, an actual decrease of
130–150 thousand has occurred.

New terms were coined in attempts to convey the properties

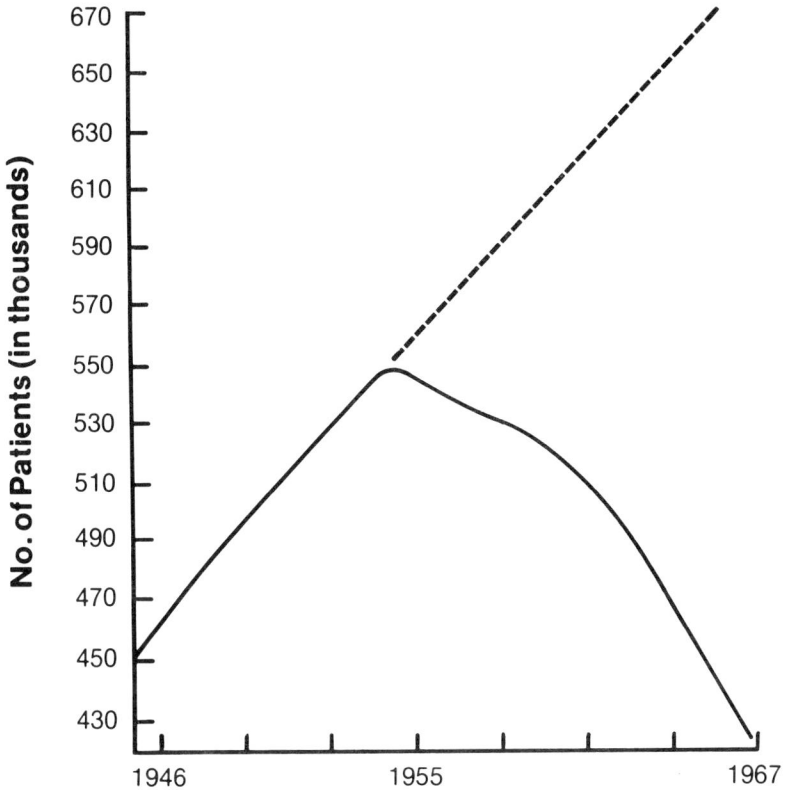

Figure 1. Number of patients in state and local government mental hospitals in the United States, 1946-1967.

of chlorpromazine and related agents and to distinguish them from older CNS depressants. Such names appeared as tranquilizers (indicating a calming effect without enforcement of sleep), ataraxics (denoting peace of mind) and neuroleptics (meaning diminution in intensity of nerve function). Until recently, *tranquilizer* had been the term most frequently used. Unfortunately, medicines prescribed for the treatment of milder psychiatric disorders, such as anxiety states, also have been called tranquilizers. Now the term *antipsychotic* usually is applied to drugs used in treating psychoses, to distinguish them from antianxiety agents.

The Discovery of Chlorpromazine

The remarkable therapeutic effects of chlorpromazine were not at all predictable. Our ignorance of the biochemical events occurring in the function and malfunction of the brain still exceeds our knowledge. No biochemical theory of mental illness guided the chemists who synthesized chlorpromazine. How, then, was this drug discovered?

Chlorpromazine evolved from a variety of individual and collective research activities spanning more than half a century of endeavor in several scientific fields. As in the discovery of many other therapeutic agents, chance observations and circumstances, such as war, played major roles. But above all, the crucial forces of discovery were the curiosity, imagination and prepared minds of chemical, biological and clinical investigators who persisted in exploring beyond the boundaries of established fact.

Chlorpromazine is a synthetic organic chemical not closely related to any of the various drugs that have been isolated from natural materials. As the structural formula illustrates, chlorpromazine contains a group of atoms called an aminoalkly sidechain attached to the nitrogen (N) atom of the central ring of the tricyclic phenothiazine ring system.

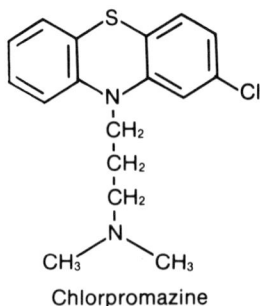

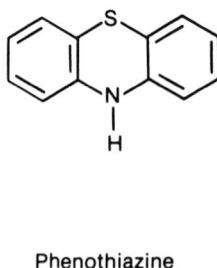

Chlorpromazine   Phenothiazine

For the origin of chlorpromazine we must look back to the latter half of the 19th century to some research achievements of the flourishing dye industry. This industry was founded in England in 1856 by W. H. Perkin who accidentally discovered that oxidation of aniline, an amino derivative of benzene, produced a beautiful purple dye called mauve. This event, of great commercial value, stimulated further experimentation in which various amines related to aniline were subjected to numerous types of chemical reactions. In this research, phenothiazine chemistry had its beginning. Unknowingly, Caro synthesized a compound containing the phenothiazine ring system when, in 1876, he heated dimethylaminoaniline with sulfur and obtained a blue dye, later named methylene blue.

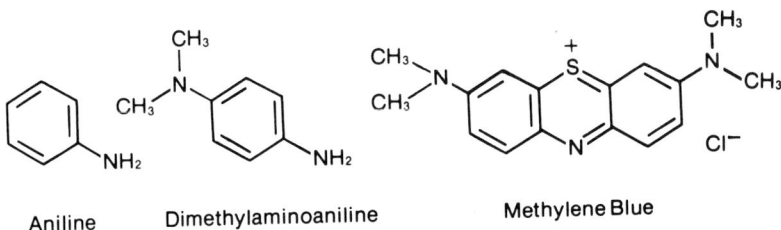

Aniline   Dimethylaminoaniline   Methylene Blue

A few years later, A. Bernthsen showed that methylene blue is a phenothiazine derivative and, in the course of his experiments, synthesized phenothiazine itself. His thorough investigations provided much of the knowledge that would be needed many decades later for the synthesis of chlorpromazine and other drugs.

Synthetic Antimalarials

A few years after Bernthsen's work, came the first sign that phenothiazine derivatives might have therapeutic value. In 1891, Paul Ehrlich, the father of chemotherapy, observed that methylene blue helped patients suffering from malaria. This was the first synthetic antimalarial agent to be discovered. But at the time no one pursued the lead provided by Ehrlich's observation. Only the demands of war some 20 years later forced further investigation.

For centuries, quinine—a constituent of the bark of the cinchona tree—had served as the chief means of treating malaria throughout the world. But during World War I the Germans found themselves cut off from the main world supply of this

naturally occurring drug and had to look for a synthetic substitute. Ehrlich's observation served as the starting point of the
search. W. Schulemann and his co-workers first synthesized
compounds related to methylene blue. One of these, a
diethylaminoethyl derivative, proved to be a more active
antimalarial than methylene blue but was too toxic to be useful.

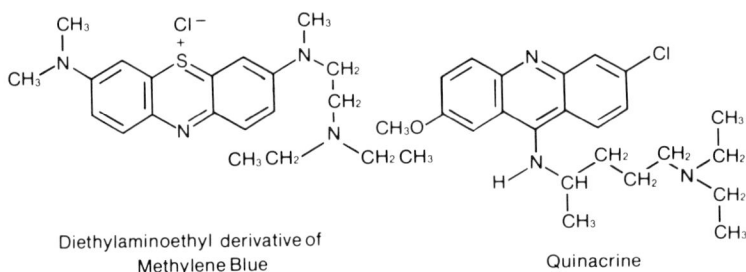

Diethylaminoethyl derivative of
Methylene Blue

Quinacrine

If you compare the structure of the phenothiazine derivative
with that of methylene blue, you will see that a methyl (CH_3)
group on one of the nitrogen atoms of methylene blue has been
replaced with an aminoalkyl group, in this case a
diethylaminoethyl group.

Although Schulemann's initial research did not provide the
medicine that the Germans were seeking, it turned out to be
crucial to the development of synthetic chemotherapeutic
agents against malaria, and other drugs as well. It led to the idea
that aminoalkyl side-chains were essential for high antimalarial
activity. Schulemann and other German chemists combined
these side-chains with many other ring systems and in due
course found a number of satisfactory antimalarials. One of
these is quinacrine, which together with quinine, enjoyed the
greatest clinical usage for many years. Once again,
phenothiazine derivatives were ignored if not forgotten until the
exigencies of war reawakened interest in them.

During World War II, as fighting raged in tropical and
subtropical countries where malaria was endemic, scientists
spurred the search for agents more effective and less toxic than
quinacrine and quinine. The quest was particularly urgent for

the Allies, because early Japanese victories in Southeast Asia in 1941 denied them access to the quinine-producing areas of the world. Many chemists, particularly in the United States and Britain, mobilized for the task. As part of the program, H. Gilman in America decided to reinvestigate the phenothiazines. Instead of methylene blue derivatives, he synthesized a group of compounds in which the aminoalkyl chains were attached to the central nitrogen atom of the phenothiazine ring. The structure below shows one of the Gilman compounds. Like quinacrine, it carries a diethylaminoalkyl side-chain.

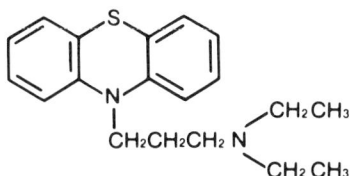

10-Aminoalkylphenothiazine

Unlike quinacrine, however, Gilman's phenothiazine derivatives were found in laboratory tests to be essentially lacking in antimalarial activity. Gilman published the negative results in 1944 in the *Journal of the American Chemical Society*. Again phenothiazine derivatives seemed destined for the scrapheap of negative or unpromising research findings. But this time, not so. By a happy coincidence some French scientists were interested in the same type of compounds, and they gave the phenothiazines another chance.

New Antihistamines

Researchers in the laboratories of the Société des Usines Chimiques Rhône-Poulenc, a French chemical and pharmaceutical company, also decided to study the same type of phenothiazines which Gilman prepared for antimalarial activity. They started their project a little later than Gilman. Fortunately, thanks to a delay in receipt of foreign scientific publications during the war, the Frenchmen did not know about Gilman's negative results. Otherwise they might not have continued their project. They confirmed that the aminoalkyl phenothiazines do not have significant antimalarial activity. But the Rhône-Poulenc scientists and their outside collaborators, such as D. Bovet at the Pasteur Institute and B. Halpern, did not dismiss the phenothiazines for lack of this activity. Instead, they pursued a variety of pharmacological actions and tested new candidate drugs for effects other than those originally expected or hoped for. In screening the phenothiazines for pharmacological activity, they soon discovered that some of the derivatives were potent antihistamines.

Rhône-Poulenc scientists had been interested in antihistamines since the late 1930s. Histamine is a chemical occurring widely in organs and tissues. Normally most of it is attached to certain cellular constituents where it is stored in a bound form, which is physiologically inert. But if released from its binding sites into tissue fluids, histamine produces profound, deleterious physiological effects. Much evidence indicates that many of the symptoms of such allergies as hay fever are due to an action of released histamine. Bovet, at the Pasteur Institute, wanted to find a drug that would antagonize the effects of histamine, and he devised animal tests to detect such an agent. In 1937, he observed antihistamine activity for the first time in some compounds synthesized years before by his colleague, E. Fourneau, which they had studied in the course of research for new antimalarials. One of these compounds was F 929 in which an aminoalkyl group is attached to a benzene ring through an oxygen atom (0). Further study revealed that the oxygen atom could be replaced with nitrogen. Compound F 1571 was a more potent antihistamine than F 929 but too toxic to be tested in man. Stimulated by Bovet's observations, chemists at Rhône-Poulenc initiated a research program to find more effective and less toxic antihistamines. After some experimentation they found that 2339 RP, named phenbenzamine, was a sufficient improvement over F 929 and F 1571 to justify clinical trial. Its introduction into the clinic, marked with great success, was a major step forward in the therapy of allergic diseases. Further research in the United States as well as France during World War II produced numerous antihistamines superior to phenbenzamine. One of these is chlorpheniramine.

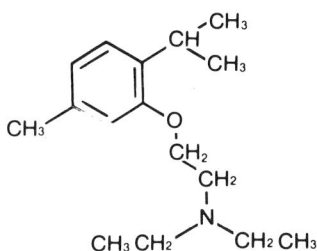

Compound F 929   Compound F 1571

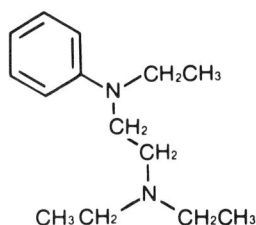

Meanwhile the Rhone-Poulenc group and their collaborators continued to search for even better antihistamines. They were struck by the long duration of action as well as high potency of one of the aminoalkyl phenothiazines—experimental compound 3277 RP, later named promethazine. It proved to be an excellent antihistamine in man and was soon introduced into medicine.

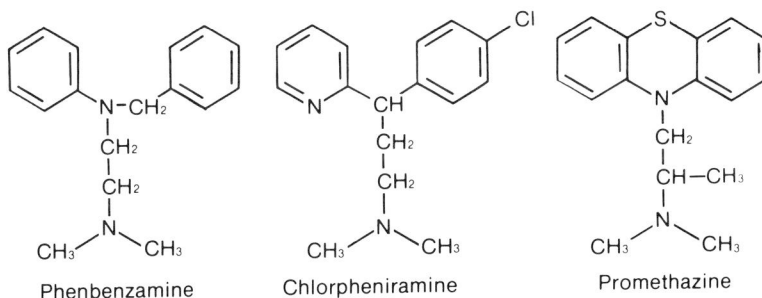

Phenbenzamine   Chlorpheniramine   Promethazine

CNS Depressant Effects

Perhaps it should not have been too surprising that a phenothiazine derivative such as promethazine possesses antihistamine activity. The molecular structures of phenbenzamine and promethazine have features in common. What was unexpected was an interesting side-effect of promethazine—a sedation much more pronounced than with other antihistamines. Meanwhile, scientists found it caused a marked prolongation of sleep induced in mice by anesthetics, and in 1950 the French surgeon H. Laborit introduced it into clinical anesthesia as a potentiating agent.

Spurred on by these signs of the CNS depressant action of promethazine, biologists and chemists at Rhône-Poulenc started a search for phenothiazine derivatives having even more pronounced CNS effects. At first they relied heavily on decrease of spontaneous movements (motor activity) and potentiation of anesthetics in animals as pharmacological tests for depressant activity. In addition to the phenothiazine derivatives that he had prepared as potential antimalarials, P. Charpentier synthesized others for study in the new research program. In December 1950, he submitted for testing experimental compound 4560 RP, later called chlorpromazine, to S. Courvoisier and her associates. They soon discovered that this compound, so similar to promethazine in molecular structure, differed markedly in its pharmacological actions.

Chlorpromazine showed a remarkable ability to decrease motor activity in animals and to prolong sleep induced by barbiturates and other anesthetics. It also effectively prevented apomorphine-induced emesis in dogs. Further studies revealed that chlorpromazine had the unusual property of selectively inhibiting learned behavior of animals. In one experimental procedure, the conditioned avoidance-escape response test, a rat is put into a box with a grid floor through which electric shocks may be delivered. (See Figure 2.)

At first, shocks are delivered at the same time a buzzer is sounded. The rat quickly learns to escape the shocks by climbing a pole suspended from the top of the box. Later the animal becomes conditioned to climb the pole in response to the buzzer only. Chlorpromazine inhibits the conditioned response to the buzzer. In other words, the drug-treated rat does not climb the pole at the sound of the buzzer, but promptly does so when shocks are delivered. Selective blockage of the conditioned response is a characteristic effect of chlorpromazine and related drugs which distinguishes them from older CNS depressants such as barbiturates. The latter, at doses sufficient to block the conditioned response, also inhibit to some extent the unconditioned response to shock. The barbiturates impair motor function in the animal so it is unable to climb the pole.

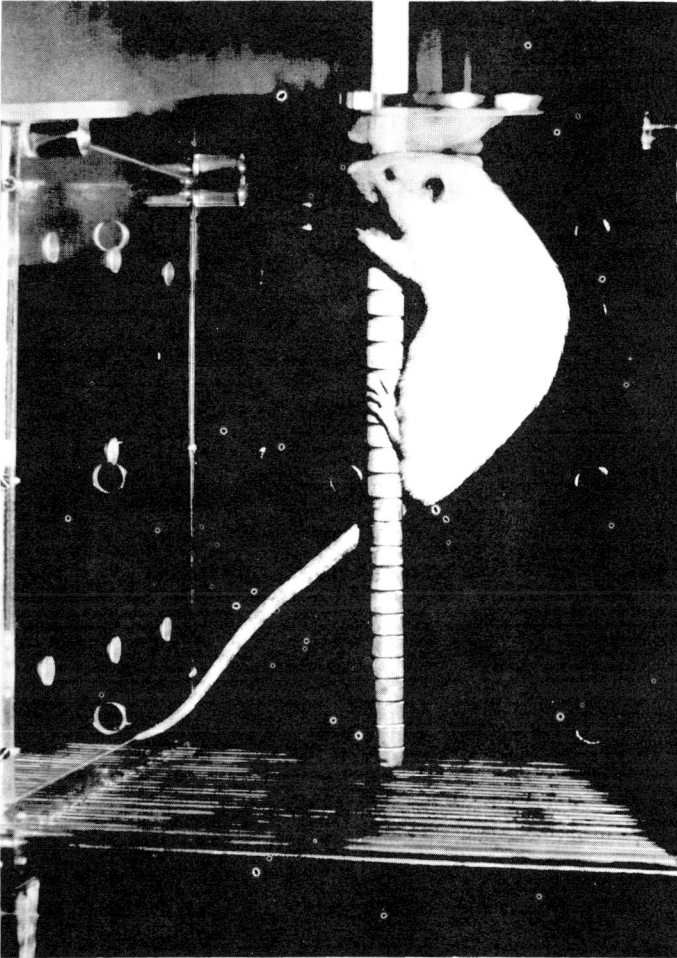

Figure 2. Conditioned avoidance-escape response test. Rat avoids shock grid floor by climbing the pole. From "Behavioral Effects of Some Pharmacological Agents" by L. Cook and E. Weidley in *Annals of the New York Academy of Sciences*, Vol. 66, Art. 3, pp. 740-752, 1957.

Treating Severe Mental Disorders

Deeply impressed with the remarkable pharmacological actions of chlorpromazine, the French researchers wanted to see what effects it would produce in man, even though the clinical utility of such an unusual drug was impossible to predict. In 1952, Laborit and his co-workers announced that administration of chlorpromazine, together with promethazine and an analgesic, induced a state of "artificial hibernation." They believed that a patient in this physical and mental state would require less anesthesia and could better withstand the stress of surgical trauma. These clinicans also observed that patients given chlorpromazine by itself did not lose consciousness but only became sleepy and showed lack of interest in what was going on. At last, some 60 years after Ehrlich first observed a clinical effect of a phenothiazine, the stage was set for the big discovery—the finding by the French psychiatrist J. Delay and his associates that a chemical, chlorpromazine, could be used to treat severe mental disorders. In addition to the case described in the beginning of our story, they soon found that other agitated, hyperactive psychotic patients benefitted from the drug.

Within two years, doctors in other countries confirmed observations of the French clinicians. Meanwhile, chlorpromazine also proved to be an effective antiemetic agent, as predicted by tests in dogs, and in 1954 it was first marketed in the United States by Smith Kline and French Laboratories as a treatment for nausea and vomiting. But its even greater usefulness in the treatment of psychotic states was quickly recognized.

Search for Antipsychotic Agents

The striking clinical success of chlorpromazine spurred a widespread search at Rhône-Poulenc and other laboratories in Europe and the United States for other antipsychotic agents. Thousands of additional phenothiazine derivatives were synthesized and tested. Charpentier and Courvoisier already had identified some of the structural features necessary for potent biological activity. The dimethylaminopropyl side chain in which the two nitrogen atoms are separated by three carbon atoms is optimal for antipsychotic and antiemetic activities. If the two nitrogens are separated by two carbons, as in promethazine, or by four carbons, activity is markedly di-

minished. Promazine (chlorpromazine without the chlorine atom at the 2-position of the ring system) retains some depressant
and antipsychotic activity but is considerably weaker than
chlorpromazine. Moving the chlorine atom of chlorpromazine
from the 2-position to any other position of the ring system
results in a great loss of potency. With knowledge of these
structure-activity relationships, chemists next concentrated on
the synthesis of phenothiazine derivatives with other substituents at the 2-position and other amino groups at the end of
the side chain. Two examples of the drugs that emerged from
this research are trifluoperazine and thioridazine.

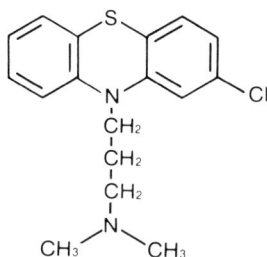

Chlorpromazine   Promethazine

These and several other phenothiazine derivatives have achieved
prominent positions in medical practice, although chlorpromazine in the 60s and early 70s remained the most widely
used antipsychotic drug throughout the world.

A comparison of the structures of trifluoperazine and
chlorpromazine reveals that the chlorine atom of the latter has
been replaced by a CF_3 called a trifluoromethyl group
(F=fluorine), and the dimethylamino group by a ring system
containing two nitrogen atoms and four carbon atoms, called a
piperazine group. Both of these structural features enhance
antipsychotic activity. Trifluoperazine, one of the most potent
phenothiazines, is 10 or more times as active as chlorpromazine.
It and certain other piperazine derivatives are important not so
much because of their high potency but because they are
"purer" antipsychotic agents than chlorpromazine.

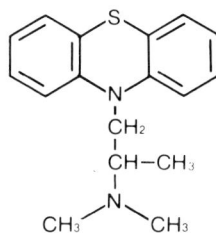

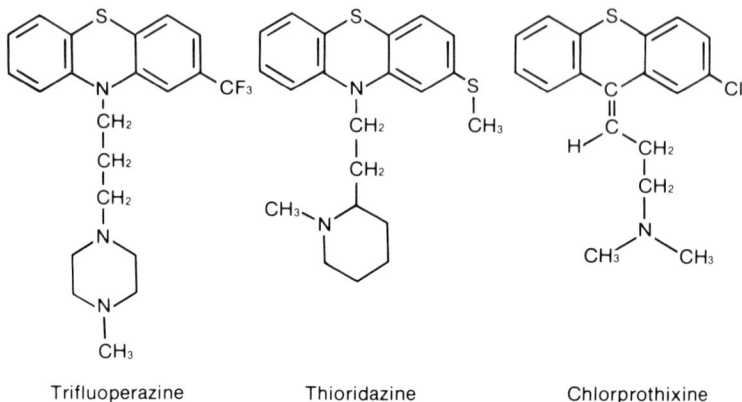

Trifluoperazine   Thioridazine   Chlorprothixine

For example, a dose of trifluoperazine which markedly decreases motor activity and blocks conditioned responses does not prolong the action of barbiturates. Thus, potentiation of anesthetics, one of the effects initially used to detect the CNS depressant actions of the phenothiazines, does not correlate with antipsychotic activity. Also, trifluoperazine produces much less sedation in man than does chlorpromazine, so this action, too, is not related to antipsychotic activity. When sedation would be detrimental to a patient, a better therapeutic effect might be obtained with trifluoperazine than with chlorpromazine. Thioridazine represents another structural modification of chlorpromazine. In addition to the SCH_3, or methylthio, group at the 2-position, this compound features a side chain in which one of the carbon atoms and the nitrogen atom of the amino group have been incorporated into a ring of six atoms. Despite this rather drastic structural change, thioridazine is about as potent an antipsychotic agent as chlorpromazine. In its structure the three carbons separate the two nitrogen atoms just as is the case in all other potent antipsychotic phenothiazines.

Although scientists quickly recognized the structural features of phenothiazine derivatives required for potent antipsychotic activity and soon discovered compounds many times more active than chlorpromazine, one vital question concerning structure-activity relationships remained. Was the phenothiazine ring system a unique requirement for antipsychotic activity? If the answer was yes, then a careful study of the chemical and physical properties of phenothiazines would help in learning their mechanism of action. But further research in various laboratories revealed that the answer was no. The phenothiazine nucleus can be replaced with certain other tricyclic systems (phenothiazine analogs). The chlorpromazine analog first found to produce potent antipsychotic activity is chlorprothixene, in which the nitrogen atom of the phenothiazine ring has been replaced by a carbon atom.

The phenothiazine ring system, therefore, is not a specific requirement for antipsychotic activity. But what chemical or physical properties do chlorpromazine and its analogs have in common that may account for their biological activity? Chemists are still seeking the answer to this question. However, if we compare the structures of chlorpromazine and its analogs with those of the antihistamines described earlier, a possible solution emerges. Many of the antihistamines, like chlorpromazine and its tricyclic analogs, have two aromatic rings attached to the atom to which the side chain is connected. But the two rings in these compounds, which lack potent antipsychotic activity, are free to rotate around the bonds that join them to the atom bearing the side chain. Much of the time the rings will be in such positions that the plane of one is approximately perpendicular to that of the other. In the antipsychotic agents the two benzene rings are tied together by a bridge of one or two atoms (forming the central ring of the tricyclic system) so that they cannot rotate very much and cannot become perpendicular to each other. As a result, molecules of the tricyclic drugs are flatter than those of the antihistamines. Perhaps certain features in the shape of a molecule are essential for antipsychotic activity. Still, the answer is not likely to be quite so simple. Among the early candidates prepared as potential antihistamines was another tricyclic compound that was to become the first of a new class of agents.

New Drugs for Mental Depression

Mental depression is not a single disease or even a well-defined group of illnesses. It is a group of symptoms in a variety of mental, emotional and physical disorders. Until the late 1950s, electroshock treatment and psychotherapy were the only generally effective means of treating severe depressions. Only a few years after discovery of the antipsychotic agents, some antidepressant drugs emerged from research on phenothiazine analogs.

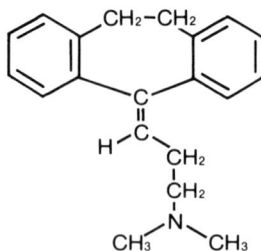

In the late 1940s, F. Hafliger, in the laboratories of J. R. Geigy, S.A., Switzerland, synthesized some aminoalkyl derivative of iminodibenzyl, a tricyclic analog of phenothiazine. It was thought that, like promethazine, these compounds might show antihistamine and sedative activities. Although some did exhibit these properties, strong interest in them developed only after the discovery in 1952 of the antipsychotic activity of chlorpromazine. During clinical studies of a few of the iminodibenzyl derivatives, R. Kuhn, in 1957, found them to be relatively ineffective in agitated patients. But he astutely observed that one compound, imipramine, appeared to be particularly beneficial in the treatment of depressive states. After further clinical studies confirmed its efficacy, imipramine was introduced as an antidepressant agent in Europe in 1958 and in the United States in 1959. Several related tricyclic antidepressives have since been developed. One of those widely used is amitriptyline.

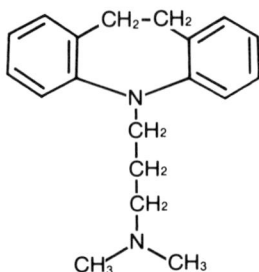

Imipramine   Amitriptyline

Thus far we have retraced the long and tortuous path that led from dyestuffs and antimalarials to the two types of drugs—the tricyclic antipsychotic and antidepressant agents—that now play major roles in the pharmacotherapy of severe psychiatric disorders. But this account would not be complete without mention of another antipsychotic agent and another group of antidepressants that, by remarkable coincidence, were discovered at almost the same time as the tricyclic derivatives.

Only a year or so after the discovery of chlorpromazine, reserpine, a structurally complex chemical isolated from the Indian plant Rauwolfia serpentina, was found to have antipsychotic as well as antihypertensive activities. As a treatment for psychoses, however, it was quickly overshadowed by the phenothiazines. Reserpine was classed as generally less effective and more difficult to control than the phenothiazine agents. It is used today primarily as an antihypertensive. (See Chapter 7.) But because of its unusual biochemical and pharmacological actions it remains one of the most studied CNS agents.

The first antidepressant, discovered a year or two before imipramine, was not a tricyclic derivative but an antitubercular drug, iproniazid, which was found to be an inhibitor of the enzyme monoamine oxidase (MAO). (The significance of this biochemical action will be mentioned later.) Iproniazid was soon replaced by several more potent MAO inhibitors, which were used extensively for a few years in the treatment of depression. Then some serious toxic effects were observed. Today imipramine and related tricyclic drugs largely have supplanted the MAO inhibitors in the clinic, although the latter are still prescribed for selected depressed patients.

Biochemistry and Mental Illness

The intriguing pharmacological and behavioral effects of all of these CNS agents—tricyclic antipsychotics and antidepressants, reserpine and MAO inhibitors—have not only challenged biologists to try to learn how they exert their actions but have also greatly stimulated studies of the biochemical processes involved in the function and malfunction of the brain. Hence these drugs have served as invaluable tools in research, leading to biochemical theories on the transmission of nerve impulses in the brain and possible causes of mental illness.

Science has known for a long time that certain chemicals transmit peripheral (outside the CNS) nerve impulses across junctions (called synapses), between neurons (nerve cells), or between a nerve ending and a tissue regulated by the nerve. One of these chemical neurotransmitters is norepinephrine, which plays an important role in the function of the *sympathetic nervous system*. (Neurotransmitters will be discussed in more detail in Chapter 7.) Biologists have felt that some of these chemicals also act in the CNS. Three that have been found in high concentration in certain areas of the brain, particularly in the lower parts (sometimes called the primitive brain) which play a role in coordination of emotional behavior, are norepinephrine, dopamine and serotonin. They commonly are called biogenic brain amines. Because of the complexity of the neuronal systems in the brain, it has not yet been possible to prove conclusively that the brain amines do act as central neurotransmitters. But considerable evidence, much of which has been derived from studies of the antipsychotics and antidepressants, lends strong support to the idea that they do serve such a function.

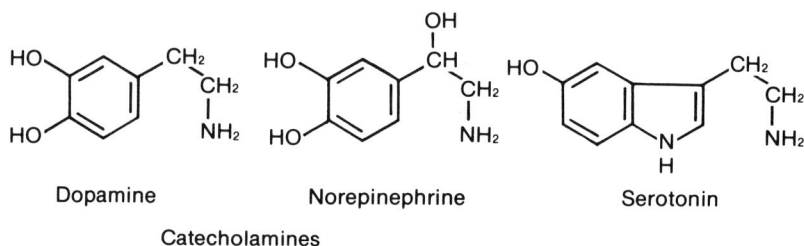

Dopamine   Norepinephrine   Serotonin

Catecholamines

The brain amines are stored in granules within the neurons. (See Figure 3 in which norepinephrine [NE] is used as an example of a brain amine.) The amines continually move in and out of the *storage granules*, and when outside they enter other small particles called *mitochondria* inside the neuron, which contain the enzyme monoamine oxidase (MAO). This enzyme catalyzes the chemical decomposition of the biogenic amines and serves to control their concentrations in the nerve cells.

The monoamine oxidase inhibitors, such as iproniazid, prevent the enzyme from destroying the amines. The result is in-

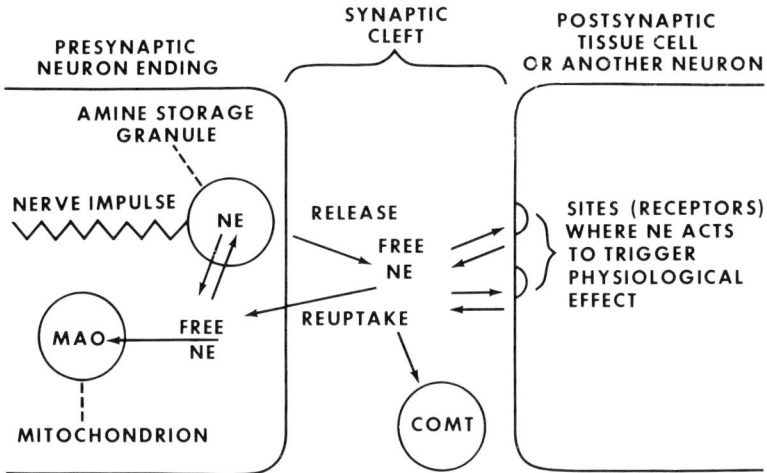

Figure 3. Schematic diagram of the adrenergic nerve terminal.

creased or decreased transmission of nerve impulses depending on whether the amines are acting as stimulatory or inhibitory transmitters.

Along with its CNS depressant and antipsychotic actions, reserpine has the remarkable ability to deplete the brain (as well as peripheral tissues) of biogenic amines. It seems to do this by blocking the mechanism for uptake of the amines into the storage granules. If the amine molecules that move out of the granules cannot return, more of them come in contact with MAO and are destroyed. Then there is a lower concentration of them in the nerve cells and, as a result, transmission of nerve impulses is altered.

If the CNS depression produced by reserpine results from a decreased concentration of one or more of the biogenic amines, it is not unreasonable to think that an increased concentration, caused by the MAO inhibitors, might produce a kind of opposite effect—an antidepressant action. Support for this idea came from an observation that reserpine, when given to animals pre-treated with iproniazid, causes excitement rather than depression. With both the destruction of the amines and their return to the storage granules blocked by the combined actions of the two drugs, very high concentrations of free neurotransmitters are produced instead of the low levels caused by reserpine alone. Such thoughts and observations inspired the clinical testing of iproniazid as a treatment of depression.

The pronounced effects of reserpine and the MAO inhibitors on the brain amine levels appeared to offer the basis for a plausible hypothesis of the biochemical mechanisms underlying antipsychotic and antidepressant activity. But biologists were baffled in their first attempts to fit chlorpromazine, imipramine and other tricyclic CNS drugs into the theoretical scheme. These drugs neither increase nor decrease concentrations of norephinephrine, dopamine or serotonin. Further search, however, indicated that their pharmacological actions may also be mediated through effects on brain amines but in ways different from those in which reserpine and the MAO inhibitors act. First evidence of this phenomenon came from studies of peripheral sympathetic nerves.

The terminal of a sympathetic neuron is separated from the tissue cell it regulates by a tiny gap called the synaptic cleft. (See Figure 3.) As the nerve impulse reaches the nerve ending, molecules of the neurotransmitter norepinephrine are released through the neuronal membrane into the cleft. They cross the cleft and briefly impinge on receptors on the tissue cell membrane to trigger a physiological effect, for example, contraction of blood vessel walls. (See Chapter 7.) Many of the norepinephrine molecules then recross the synaptic cleft and enter the nerve ending where they are ready to be released by the next nerve impulse. Those molecules that do not return to the neuron are rapidly destroyed by an enzyme having the long name catechol-O-methyltransferase (COMT), which is present in the synaptic cleft or near the norepinephrine receptors of the tissue cells.

In her early studies, Courvoisier noted that chlorpromazine inhibits some peripheral effects of norepinephrine. Evidently it prevents the biogenic amine from occupying postsynaptic tissue receptors. Later, imipramine was found to enhance peripheral actions of norepinephrine. This seems to be due to blockade of a norepinephrine concentrating mechanism at the nerve mem brane. The result is that reuptake of the neurotransmitter is diminished. Consequently, a greater amount remains ready for action in the vicinity of the amine receptors.

It is postulated that the tricyclic drugs act on the CNS through analogous mechanisms. A prevalent view is that these agents interfere with the catecholamines, norephinephrine and dopamine, in their role as CNS neurotransmitters. At junctions (synapses) of nerve cells, these amines are released from the terminal of one neuron, cross the synaptic cleft and impinge on amine receptors of another neuron, thus transmitting the nerve impulse from one cell to another. Chlorpromazine produces its effects through blockade of the postsynaptic amine receptors, and imipramine through inhibiting reuptake of norepinephrine by the presynaptic nerve ending. According to these postulates, the antidepressant action of imipramine and the MAO inhibitors may be due to a common biochemical effect of the two types of drugs produced by different mechanisms. Both types of drugs may cause an increase in concentration of norephinephrine at its receptors—the MAO inhibitors by preventing destruction of the amine in the nerve cell, making more available for release into the synaptic cleft, and imipramine by inhibiting reuptake of the amine from the cleft to the presynaptic nerve ending.

Parkinsonism

We still lack conclusive evidence that a malfunction of neurotransmitters occurs in psychotic and depressive states. The roles played by any one or all of the biogenic amines and the postulated mechanisms of action of the CNS drugs remain to be established. But the hypotheses have provided an important basis for extensive research, which continues today. From studies of the biogenic brain amines has come a new drug for the treatment of Parkinson's disease or parkinsonism, a severe neurological ailment.

Symptoms of parkinsonism are muscular rigidity and tremors caused by a malfunction in the *basal ganglia*, neural systems in the CNS. The concentration of dopamine in the basal ganglia of patients with parkinsonism is significantly below normal. This suggests that administration of dopamine would compensate for the deficiency, but the amine when given orally does not enter the CNS. However, its natural precursor, dopa (dihydroxyphenylalanine), a chemical that is converted to dopamine by an enzyme in nerve cells, can enter the CNS. Administration of dopa has caused marked improvement in many parkinsonism patients. Dopa is now recognized to be generally superior to other medications for the treatment of Parkinson's disease.

Some of the most characteristic side effects produced by reserpine and the tricyclic antipsychotic agents are symptoms that closely resemble those of parkinsonism. The observation that dopamine levels are low in the basal ganglia of parkinsonism patients lends further support to the idea that these drugs interfere with neurotransmitters in the brain. Reserpine depletes dopamine in the basal ganglia. Perhaps chlorpromazine blocks postsynaptic dopamine receptors so that the amine cannot transmit the nerve impulse.

Although the antipsychotic and antidepressant agents are mainly the products of empirical research and serendipity, knowledge and theories of the mechanism of action promise new, rational approaches to the discovery of better medicines for treating psychiatric disorders.

In the meantime, will further research on antimalarials again lead to other unexpected CNS agents as it did in the case of the phenothiazines? Probably not, but at this moment a chemist may be synthesizing a new compound, perhaps a potential diuretic or anti-inflammatory drug, that will start the whole surprising, fascinating process over again.

Suggested Reading

Asimov, I. *The Human Brain: Its Capacities and Functions.* New York: New American Library, 1965.

Burger, A. (Ed.) *Medicinal Chemistry.* (3rd ed.) New York: Interscience Publishers, 1970.

Burger, A. (Ed.) Drugs Affecting the Central Nervous System. *Medicinal Research Monographs,* New York: Marcel Dekker, Inc. 1968, 2.

Goodman, L. S., & Gilman, A. (Eds.) *The Pharmacological Basis of Therapeutics.* (4th ed.) New York: MacMillan, 1970.

Gordon, M. (Ed.) Psychopharmacological Agents. *Medicinal Chemistry,* New York: Academic Press, 1964 and 1967, *4* (1, 2).

Gould, R. F. (Ed.) Molecular Modification in Drug Design. *Advances in Chemistry,* American Chemical Society, Washington, 1964, No. 45.

McGaugh, J. L., Weinberger, N. M., & Whalen, R. E. (Eds.) *Psychobiology: The Biological Bases of Behavior* (Readings from Scientific American). San Francisco: W. H. Freeman and Company, 1966.

Shideman, F. E. (Ed.) *Take as Directed—Our Modern Medicines.* Cleveland, Ohio: The Chemical Rubber Co., 1967.

CHAPTER 6

Hormones and Control of Body Functions

Hershel L. Herzog

In 1904 at the University of London, Ernest Bayliss and William Starling were investigating the flow of a digestive juice from the pancreas into the upper end of the small intestine. The juice flowed only in response to the entry of stomach contents into the intestine. They asked the question, "What gives the signal that makes the juice begin to flow?"

Up to this time scientists had believed that the message was carried by nerves connecting the intestine with the pancreas. Bayliss and Starling cut all of these nerves in an animal and showed that the juice still flowed in response to a meal. They then separated the mucous membrane of the intestine, mixed it with some stomach acid and injected this preparation into the bloodstream of a test animal. They found that the pancreatic juice flowed even in the absence of food.

Bayliss and Starling concluded that a substance forms in response to action of stomach acid on the intestinal lining. This substance, or hormone as they called it (from the Greek *hormao*, meaning "I excite"), was then carried by the blood to the pancreas, where it gave a signal to secrete. The two scientists called the intestinal hormone secretin.

These experiments gave the first clear proof that chemical messengers trigger remote biological events—a discovery that was to make possible the development of many new classes of medicines. In this chapter we trace the history of important ideas emanating from such discoveries.

The external effects of hormone insufficiency had been recognized in ancient times. Castration of human beings produced eunuchoid characteristics, such as obesity, freedom from facial hair and absence of libido. Slaves were sometimes castrated to make them safer guards for the female members of households. Castration was also used to preserve the soprano voice in the male (soprano castrato) for performance of opera and song at a time when theater life was considered unsuitable for women. Gelded horses and bulls were docile and thus better suited for work in transportation and agriculture. The caponized cock described in Gesner's *Historia Animalum* (1555) looked and behaved like a hen—it was combless and did not crow or fight. Capon flesh was fatter and more appetizing than that of the scrawny rooster.

Scientists failed to relate these effects to chemical agents secreted by the male sex glands until long after the first published scientific studies from which such inferences might have been drawn were conducted in 1849 by Arnold Berthold, a professor of zoology at Gottingen University. Berthold showed that cocks whose testes had been relocated in their abdomens retained their male characteristics. Autopsies of these cocks revealed that blood circulation had been spontaneously reestablished between the testes and the abdominal wall after transplantation. He concluded that testes acted in some way on the blood, which in turn acted on the organism as a whole. Unfortunately, this pioneering observation, which should have pointed to the existence of hormones, was neglected by the world of science until 1910, when Berthold's publication was rediscovered.

Thyroxine—Hormone of the Thyroid

Happily, when circumstances are right for an idea they speak to the minds of many men. In 1873, a cretinoid disease of middle aged women characterized by dimming mental acuity, a puffy waterlogged appearance and loss of hair was described for the first time by William Gull of Guy's Hospital in London. This condition was later called myxoedema. At about the same time, Swiss physicians began treating goiter surgically by removing large parts of the thyroid gland. In mountainous areas potable waters tend to contain little or no iodine, and their exclusive use by man often leads to this deficiency disease, which is marked by gross enlargement of the thyroid.

Jacques Reverdin, professor of surgery at Geneva, observed that among patients subjected to thyroidectomy, a substantial number developed cachexia strumipriva, a condition resembling myxoedema. In 1882, he concluded that the two ailments were one and the same. Soon thereafter, Felix Semon, a German physician practicing in London, suggested that both diseases were caused by loss of function of the thyroid gland. Subsequent laboratory testing on the effects of thyroidectomy on monkeys and other species verified this hypothesis.

George Redmayne Murray, a professor of pathology at Durham, England, then leaped to the conclusion that myxoedema might be treated with an extract of thyroid gland. In 1891, he reported control of myxoedema in a 46-year-old woman through continuing administration of a glycerine extract of sheep thyroid. *This experiment, a landmark in chemotherapy, represented the first successful use of hormonal agents to treat disease.*

Murray did not know exactly what chemical material in the injected mixture was responsible for his therapeutic success. Eventually, at the Mayo Foundation on Christmas day, 1914, Edward Kendall, who later shared the Nobel Prize for his work on cortisone, isolated the active principle of the thyroid gland as a pure crystalline substance. He called it thyroxine. Its precise chemical structure, established by Harington in 1926, is shown below.

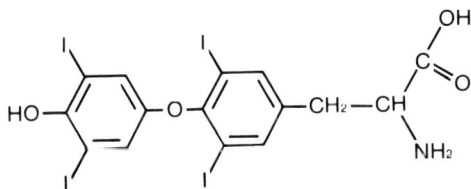

Figure 1. Thyroxine—hormone of the thyroid.

Investigators had determined much earlier that the thyroid gland requires a dietary source of iodine, and the reason is apparent from the high iodine content of thyroxine. With the structure known, it became possible to prepare the hormone by synthetic means. Today, both chemically synthesized thyroxine and dried bovine thyroid gland, a byproduct of the slaughter-house, are used in thyroid replacement therapy.

Kendall was not the first to show that it was possible to isolate from glandular material discrete chemical entities that could mimic some or all the physiological effects of the gland.

Adrenal Hormones

In 1894, George Oliver and Edward Schafer at University College, London, found that intravenous injection of an extract of medulla (core) of the canine adrenal gland raised a dog's blood pressure. By 1897, John J. Abel and Albert Crawford at Johns Hopkins University had separated from adrenal tissue a crystalline material that they believed was the adrenal hormone.

Actually, the procedure of isolation had changed the hor-mone. Later, in 1901, Jokichi Takamine, and independently, Thomas Aldrich, modified the Abel-Crawford procedure and unmasked a true adrenal hormone, now called adrenaline or epinephrine. Fortuitously, the Abel-Crawford artifact also raised canine blood pressure, as did crystalline epinephrine. Late in 1904, a Hoechst scientist, Friedrich Stolz, proved the correct structure by preparing the hormone with simple chemical reagents—without the intervention of living tissue.

Knowledge of structure is the chemist's most powerful tool in designing new and improved medicines. One of the earliest ex-amples of structural innovation came from knowledge of epinephrine. George Barger and Henry Dale in 1910 described a study of the blood pressure elevating effects of a series of amines (compounds possessing an atom of nitrogen), many of which contained the peculiar and special beta-phenylethylamine skeleton present in epinephrine. (See Figure 2). From this study they discovered that maximum pressor activity was associated with compounds that, like epinephrine, bore the beta-phenylethylamine unit.

In subsequent evaluation by many laboratories, epinephrine was demonstrated to stimulate the heart, giving it more forceful contractions, rapid beat and greater output. Epinephrine also constricts many blood vessels (but not the coronary vessels or

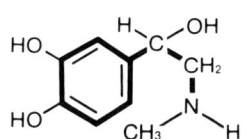

Epinephrine

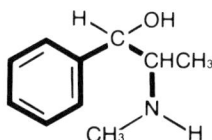

Ephedrine

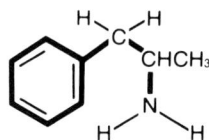

Amphetamine

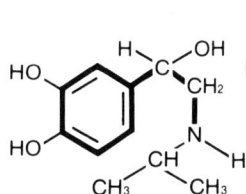

Isoproterenol

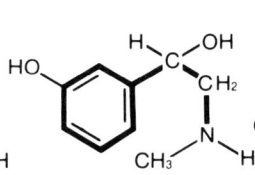

Phenylephrine

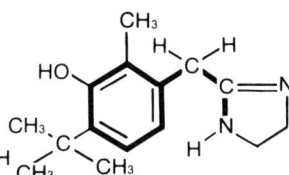

Oxymetazoline

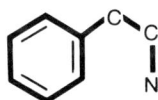

Beta-phenylethylamine Skeleton

Figure 2. The common theme of adrenergic drugs.

muscular arterioles). It stimulates respiration, elevates blood sugar, relaxes pulmonary bronchioles and dilates the pupil of the eye. These actions are brought about after injection of the drug, but not after its oral administration, which limits its convenient application. Nonetheless, the physician employs epinephrine to combat shock and extreme fatigue. It also relieves asthmatic attacks (relaxes bronchioles), reduces nasal congestion (constricts blood vessels of the nose and displaces fluid from the engorged nasal mucosa), lowers appetite and increases alertness or wakefulness. Unfortunately, a patient cannot use the agent with comfort (or in cases of associated heart disease, with safety) because of undesirable effects on his heart and blood pressure. Hence the use of epinephrine largely has been restricted to treatment of shock and a few other acute indications.

Synthetic Analogs

Recognition of these potentially valuable properties of epinephrine led to a search for drugs that would possess some of the desirable attributes but would be relatively free of cardiac and pressor effects. The beta-phenylethylamine structural unit has been a recurring chemical theme in the quest for such compounds. Eventually, researchers found safer, more convenient and more selective agents for treating the wide variety of ailments on which epinephrine has favorable effects. The major discoveries, many of which are illustrated in Figure 2, contain without exception the beta-phenylethylamine skeleton. By subtle structural alteration it has been possible to enhance favorable and diminish unfavorable actions of epinephrine.

For example, ephedrine, an alkaloid extracted from the ancient Chinese botanical drug Ma Huang, was shown by Chen to resemble epinephrine in its pharmacodynamic properties. Most important, it is long acting when taken by mouth (epinephrine is short acting and effective only by injection); it is stable for long periods in dosage forms (epinephrine is quite labile); and it is less toxic. Extensively used to treat hay fever and mild asthma, ephedrine is produced readily by chemical synthesis, so its botanical origins concern only the historian.

Amphetamine, a synthetic drug not found in nature, was discovered by G. Alles in 1927 to be a useful stimulant; when taken by mouth, it induces alertness and wakefulness and combats depression. It, too, has less pressor activity and toxicity than epinephrine. An associated effect of amphetamine is appetite depression. As part of a regimen involving reduced food intake, it has been useful in treatment of obesity. In more recent times, unfortunately, habitual users have misused amphetamine and related drugs for their stimulant actions to obtain kicks to help them escape from the more depressing aspects of daily life. Consequently, drug abuse laws have been passed to control the production and use of such agents.

The synthetic drugs phenylephrine and oxymetazoline when applied topically in the nose as drops or spray, combat the nasal congestion symptoms of colds or allergies. Doses required by this route of administration are so minute that they have no observable effects on heart rate or blood pressure. Single doses of oxymetazoline often are effective for as long as eight hours.

Isoproterenol, another product of the laboratory, is prescribed often for asthma. Inhaled directly into the lungs, the drug acts on constricted bronchioles. It is not free of cardiac and pressor actions, but its convenience and effectiveness have made it a successful product.

The detailed knowledge of chemical structure and biological functions of a natural hormone (epinephrine) have encouraged development of a wide variety of synthetic drugs of specific chemical design and selective biological action. The pharmaceutical industry is pursuing continued and intensive study of structure and function with conspicuous success in the development of new drugs.

Complex Mammalian Hormones

Knowledge about hormones other than those of the thyroid and adrenal medulla has developed more slowly because of the problems of isolation from other endocrine organs and the complex structures of the chemical agents thus obtained. We now classify the organs tabulated in Table 1 as endocrine, in that they are known to produce agents that are transported by the blood to a remote tissue where they act to influence some vital chemicobiological processes.

Hormones fall into four major chemical classes: phenol, steroid, polypeptide and protein. Each class involves a characteristic molecular structure. It is only through the precise fixing of structure that integrity and function of each of the hormones are maintained. Changes in the arrangement or number of atoms often are sufficient to cancel or alter in a surprising way the biological effects of the resulting modified hor-

mones. We have already seen that analogs (related structures) of
the simple phenolic hormone, epinephrine, can retain elements
of the activity of the parent, even though the degree of structural change appears quite extensive.

Early Discoveries in Steroid Chemistry

Steroid hormones are also subject to structural manipulation
with remarkable and sometimes beneficial effect. However, the
elements of structure required for hormonal activity in this class
seem to be somewhat more precisely drawn by nature than
those for the simple phenolic hormones.

Scientific understanding of steroid hormones also began in
the 19th century. At first biology and organic chemistry, still in
their infancy, made scant progress toward the isolation and
description of the hormonal agents that control the sex characteristics of the male. During this period workers in the medi-
cochemical fields became aware that a whole class of powerful
regulatory agents was formed in exceedingly minute amounts
by many of the body's glands. They recognized that to isolate
and identify a hormonal agent of unknown chemical properties
from a large amount of biological material, like glands or urine,
it would be necessary to determine the degree of enrichment of
the active principle following application of separation techniques.

In the history of research on the male hormone, the next step
following the early work of Berthold was taken by A. Pezard,
who reported in 1911 that testicular material injected into a
capon would cause the comb to regenerate. By 1929, Thomas
Gallagher and Fred Koch, working at the University of Chicago,
had developed this observation into a quantitative tool for determining the male hormone content of concentrates from
fractionation of bull testes. Application of the same bioassay to
male human urine demonstrated the presence of small but
measurable levels of male hormone-like substance.

About this time Adolph Butenandt at Göttingen received a
generous gift of the concentrate from about 4,000 gallons of

Table 1. Some important mammalian hormones—description, source and functions.

Endocrine Organ	Major Hormone	Biological Function	Chemical Class
1. Adrenals a. cortex	hydrocortisone	to combat stress; to conserve the body salt and water	steroid
	aldosterone	to conserve the body salt and water	steroid
b. medulla	epinephrine	to combat stress	simple phenolic β-phenethylamine
2. Duodenal mucosa	secretin	to promote digestion of food by stimulating release of digestive enzymes	polypeptide
3. Gonads a. testes	testosterone	to stimulate development of male sex character and behavior	steroid
b. ovaries	estradiol progesterone	to stimulate development of female sex character and behavior; to control events leading to reproduction (i.e. ovulation, fertilization, implantation)	steroid steroid
4. Pancreas	insulin glucagon	to stimulate utilization of sugar by tissues to stimulate release of sugar from liver	polypeptide polypeptide
5. Parathyroid	parathyroid hormone	to help regulate calcium and phosphorus content of bones and blood by causing release of calcium and phosphorus from bone	protein
6. Pituitary	ACTH[1] FSH[2] LH[3]	to stimulate hydrocortisone production in adrenal to stimulate growth and release of egg from ovary to stimulate sperm production; stimulate testosterone (male) and estradiol (female) production by gonads	polypeptide protein protein
	oxytocin	to stimulate uterine contraction and milk flow in pregnancy	polypeptide
7. Placenta	chorionic gonadotrophin	to stimulate progesterone production by corpus luteum of ovary; maintenance of pregnancy	protein
8. Thyroid	thyroxine	to stimulate oxygen consumption by tissues	phenolic amino acid
	calcitonin	to help regulate calcium and phosphorus content of bones and blood by causing deposition of calcium and phosphorus into bone	polypeptide

[1] adrenocorticotrophic hormone
[2] follicle stimulating hormone
[3] luteinizing hormone

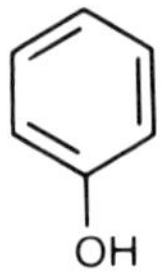

Phenol 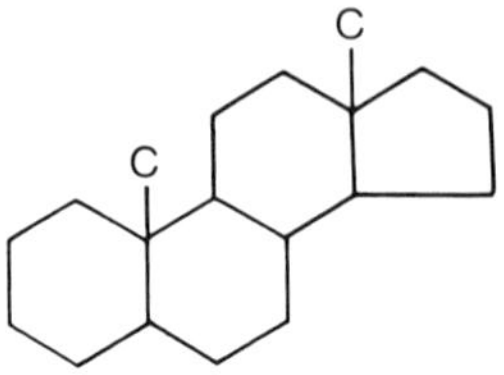   Steroid

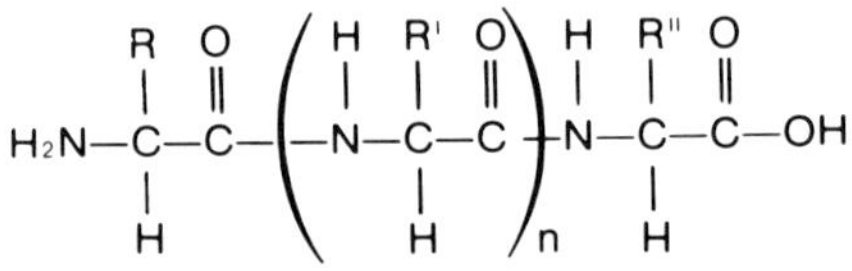

Polypeptide

Figure 3. Major chemical classes of hormones. The structure below depicts the polypeptides and proteins in which R, R' and R'' are substituents of the amino acids. An average size protein has 300 peptide units. See also Figure 9.

male urine provided by Schering-Kahlbaum, a German pharmaceutical firm. Using the new bioassay as an analytical tool, Butenandt, after prodigious labors, isolated, in 1931, a total of 15 mg. (0.0005 ounce) of a crystalline male hormone substance. He recognized that these few crystals belonged to the organic chemical class of steroids, and he correctly inferred the exact chemical structure in 1932, the same year that the basic structure of the steroid class itself was first fixed. Butenandt named his hormone androsterone.

There continued to be some speculation that the male hormone isolated from urine would not necessarily be the same as that elaborated in the organ of actual production. In studies with castrated rats and capons, E. Laquer of Amsterdam showed that testicular extracts could provide a material of even greater male hormone potency than androsterone. From 220

pounds of bull testes he isolated, in 1935, 10 mg. of a crystalline substance he called testosterone. This agent was 10 times
more powerful than androsterone in promoting comb growth.
He had identified the true male hormone. Much later investigators showed that some of the naturally produced testosterone is changed into androsterone by the liver and is then
excreted in the urine.

For a time many believed that use of male hormone could
keep men "eternally" young and virile, and the popular press
and science writers toyed with this theme at great length.
Natural production of testosterone begins to decline in most
men during their 50s, but it was hoped that the dwindling supply could be supplemented by synthetic hormone. The available
supply of bull testes could produce testosterone for no more
than a few men, so researchers devised methods of manufacture
from readily available raw materials (cholesterol from the brain
and spinal cords of cattle).

It turned out that testosterone can to some extent delay the
aging process, enhance libido and increase potency. It also
stimulates building of protein and consequent maintenance of
muscle mass and physical strength. However, there is a price to
pay for this limited rejuvenation. Testosterone encourages the
growth of the prostate gland to the extent that urination may
be seriously impeded. The remedy for an enlarged prostrate is
surgical removal of a portion of the gland. A matter of graver
concern is that the use of testosterone also increases the risk of
cancerous (as opposed to benign) growth of the prostate. For
this life-threatening condition, surgery provides no certain cure.
In spite of these risks, testosterone in one or another of its
various forms (See Figure 4) is still used to some degree in aging
males, but more often as a supplement in hormone-deficient
young men.

Female Sex Hormones

While the male hormone turned out to have great academic
interest but not much lasting medical impact, investigation of

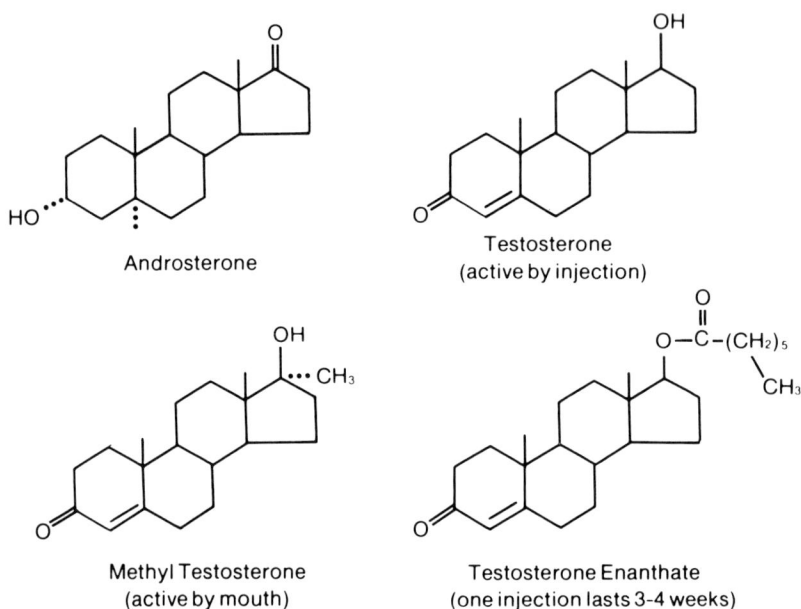

Androsterone

Testosterone
(active by injection)

Methyl Testosterone
(active by mouth)

Testosterone Enanthate
(one injection lasts 3-4 weeks)

Figure 4. Natural and synthetic androgenic steroid hormones.

the female hormone led to a revolution. Up to a point, understanding of the two classes of female sex hormones, the estrogenic and the progestational, followed the same path as that of
the male hormone. E. Knauer of Vienna showed in 1896 that
ovaries controlled the development of the female sex character
in animals by transplanting these glands into castrates, para-
phrasing A. Berthold's earlier experiment with cock testes. C. R.
Stockard and G. N. Papanicolaou of Cornell demonstrated that
the surface cells of the vagina in small mammals (e.g., mice)
undergo characteristic changes under the influence of estrogenic
hormones during each phase of estrus (heat). This principle was
later developed into a quantitative method for the assay of
estrogenic activity. When S. Aschheim and B. Zondek discovered, in 1927, that the urine of pregnant women is rich in
estrogenic substance, the next step became feasible—the isolation of a female hormone. The crystalline hormone, estrone,
was isolated by both Doisy and Butenandt in 1931. (See Figure

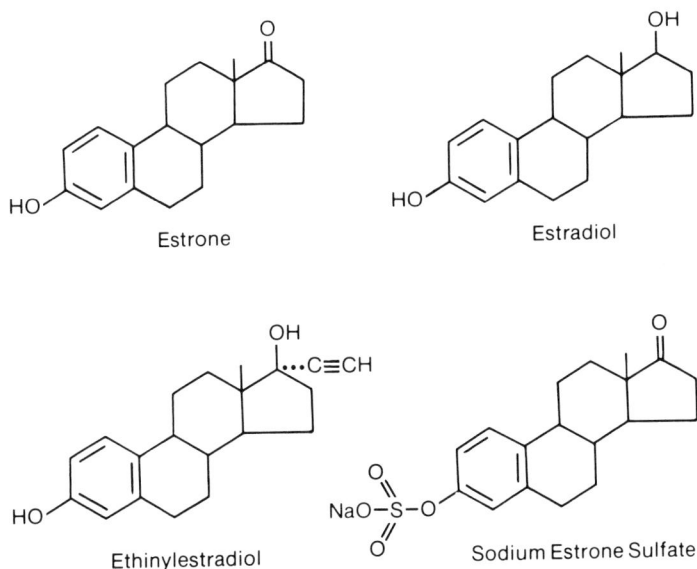

Figure 5. Natural and synthetic estrogenic steroid hormones.

5.) These scientists and several other groups established the structure of estrone in 1935.

The chemical modification of estrone into more active estrogens was begun in 1933 before its structure was completely known. The first successful derivative, estradiol, achieved through the work of E. Schwenk and F. Hildebrandt of Schering-Kahlbaum, was later shown to be present in ovarian tissue. An exceedingly powerful, orally active estrogen, ethinyl estradiol, was prepared in 1938. This compound assumed great importance in the later development of the sex hormone field.

In the early post-discovery days, and for about 20 years thereafter, estrone, estradiol, ethinylestradiol and, most prominently, a mixture of conjugated equine estrogens, were used as estrogen replacement in post-menopausal women. The last named and most widely employed product was manufactured from the urine of pregnant mares; the mixture thus obtained consisted principally of sodium estrone sulfate and several other estrogen sulfates of closely related structure.

At the same time knowledge began to accumulate about the progestational hormone of the corpus luteum, a yellow-pigmented ovarian tissue which forms after the ripening and rupture of the follicle from which the ovum springs. Fraenkel had shown in 1903 that removal of the corpus luteum of a rabbit shortly after ovulation terminates or prevents a pregnancy. G. W. Corner and W. M. Allen in 1928 demonstrated that extracts of corpus luteum can supply hormonal elements essential to pregnancy maintenance to an already pregnant rabbit from which the corpus luteum had been removed. It thus became possible to develop an assay for progestational activity, and work began on the isolation of the crystalline hormone of the corpus luteum. In 1934, groups in four laboratories, two German, one Swiss and one American, all reported success. The Butenandt group used the ovaries of 50,000 sows to prepare 20 mg. of the pure hormone, progesterone. Its chemical structure was deduced soon thereafter.

Following elucidation of structure, and development of methods of manufacture, progesterone and other steroidal agents acting like it were tried in attempts to maintain pregnancy in women prone to abortion. Since it is difficult to prove such a desired effect, this application has had limited use.

Hormones and Contraception

However, the most important chapter in the story of the female hormones was yet to come. In 1950, the medical director of the Planned Parenthood Foundation, Abraham Stone, persuaded Gregory Pincus, co-director of the Worcester Foundation for Biological Research, to try to develop a method of human contraception that would be 100 percent effective, esthetically acceptable, safe, reversible and simple to use. No small order!

At this time it was known from the work of A. W. Makepeace, G. L. Weinstein, and M. H. Friedman (University of Pennsylvania, 1937) that progesterone administered by injection to rabbits, inhibited ovulation. Pincus and his collaborator, M. C. Chang, began their experiments by feeding rabbits large doses of progesterone. The treated rabbits mated but did not ovulate. It now appeared possible that a pill might be devised which women could take to prevent pregnancy. Pincus then sought the assistance of John Rock, professor of gynecology at Harvard, to test the ability of progesterone to actually prevent ovulation in women. Twenty-seven subjects, all of whom ovulated normally, participated in various aspects of these tests. After massive doses of progesterone by mouth, 23 of the women failed to ovulate!

This experiment proved for the first time that chemical contraception was worthy of intensive study. However, three serious problem remained: (a) the efficiency of ovulation inhibition had to be 99-100 percent; (b) the cost of the drug had to be at economically attractive levels; and (c) the occasional breakthrough bleeding (bleeding between times of normal menstrual flow) had to be eliminated. To achieve these goals, Pincus solicited new and more powerful progestational compounds from G. D. Searle, a Chicago-based pharmaceutical firm and long-time supporter of Worcester Foundation activities. With knowledge of the structures of recognized progestational compounds, Frank Colton at Searle prepared a number of novel variants, which then were tested on animals. Those compounds that showed promising progestational activity went to Pincus and Chang for further study. Thus **they discovered that norethynodrel (See Figure 6) was at least 10 times more** potent in laboratory animals than progesterone. In a subsequent clinical trial with 50 women, conducted by Rock, a 10 mg. dose of norethynodrel from day 5 to day 24 of a woman's menstrual cycle suppressed ovulation with virtually 100 percent efficiency. Yet when the drug was withdrawn, normal ovulation resumed. This experiment demonstrated that ovulation control in human beings could be achieved reliably at relatively modest cost.

It later developed that the norethynodrel used in early trials contained, as an impurity, a very small amount of a powerful estrogen, mestranol (a derivative of ethinylestradiol described earlier). This fortuitous companion substance contributed to the efficacy of the preparation; it also prevented the occasional

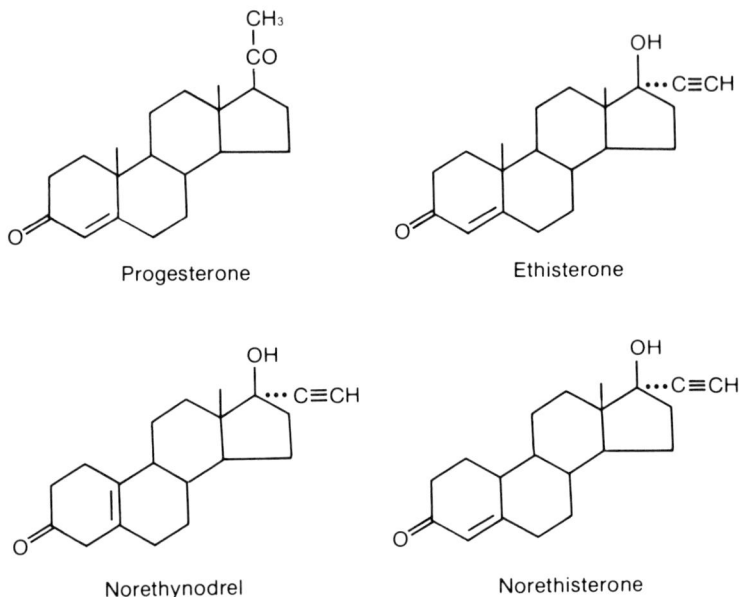

Figure 6. Ovulation inhibiting steroids.

spotting (breakthrough bleeding) associated with pure norethynodrel.

In extensive field trials begun in 1956 in Puerto Rico, the
Searle Company provided a carefully standardized mixture of
9.85 milligrams of norethynodrel and 0.15 milligrams of
mestranol as active ingredients in each tablet. Over a period of
four years more than 1,600 women participated in these trials,
contributing an exposure to pregnancy of about 3,000 woman

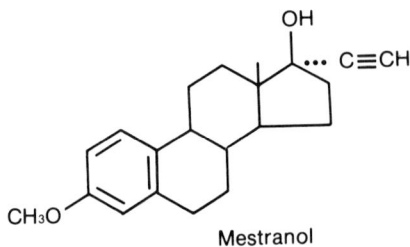

Mestranol

years. Only 45 pregnancies were recorded during the test (instead of the normal expectation of about 3,000), and many of these resulted from failure to take the drug as directed. This experiment proved unequivocally that it was possible to prevent conception in a statistically reliable way by using a chemical contraceptive technique that was comprehensible and acceptable to women in a relatively unsophisticated population. The Searle Company received approval to market this anticonceptive drug in the United States in 1960; its reliability has long since been confirmed through millions of patient-year exposures. Chemical contraception attained wide medical and social acceptance in the 60s as a most effective birth control system.

Since 1960, further research sponsored by pharmaceutical firms has contributed to development of even smaller doses of a variety of different ovulation-inhibiting anticonceptives. Reduced dosage eliminates most side effects, such as nausea and weight gain experienced by some users of earlier forms of "the pill." In addition, researchers pursue knowledge and techniques in chemical contraception by means other than inhibition of ovulation, and this avenue holds much promise for the future

Hormones of the Adrenal Cortex

Our brief history of hormone research now turns back to one of its most complicated, yet most fruitful stages. In 1855, William Addison of Guy's Hospital, London, described a fatal, wasting disease (now called Addison's disease) which was accompanied by atrophy of the adrenals. He attributed the symptoms, including anemia, feebleness of the heart and eventual death to malfunction of these glands. In 1894, E. A. Shafer and G. Oliver showed that the adrenal medulla secreted a substance which proved to be epinephrine. It was then believed that the medulla was the center of important adrenal hormone synthesis and that the adrenal cortex (bark) had no significant biological function.

This notion was overthrown in 1927 by Julius Rogoff and George Stewart at Western Reserve University. They confirmed that removal of the adrenals from dogs invariably results in

death within about two weeks. Their research also showed for
the first time that an extract of the canine adrenal cortex could
sustain life in the adrenalectomized dog for as long as 78 days.
These observations later (1934) became the basis for a bioassay
of life-maintaining activity of adrenocortical extracts devised by
J. J. Pfiffner, W. W. Swingle, and H. M. Vars at Princeton
University.

Using this and related bioassay techniques, Oscar Wintersteiner at Columbia University, E. C. Kendall at the Mayo
Foundation and T. Reichstein at the Technical University in
Zürich began intensive studies to isolate the hormones of the
adrenal cortex. By 1943, through the combined efforts of these
laboratories, 28 compounds of the steroid structural class had
been isolated in minute amounts from beef and hog adrenals.
Six of these had some degree of biological activity, either to
sustain life or to make animals more efficient in the performance of work. The six active compounds are illustrated in
Figure 7. In addition, the structures of almost all 28 were
delineated in all their marvelous complexity and detail.

It was recognized early that desoxycorticosterone, a compound that could maintain life in adrenalectomized dogs and
rats, might do the same for the relatively few sufferers of Addison's disease. And this did turn out to be the case.
Desoxycorticosterone, possessing the simplest structure of all of
the corticosteroids, is readily available through chemical
synthesis. Addison's disease also has been treated successfully
with adrenal extracts from animal sources.

The Quest for Synthetic Methodology

The other active corticosteroids were much less accessible,
because adequate chemical technology had not yet been developed. To aid in the exploration of other possible applications
of these intriguing compounds, the National Research Council
(USA) in 1942 authorized a multigroup quest for the required
synthetic methodology. Teams at Yale (under W. Bergmann),
University of Chicago (T. F. Gallagher), Mayo Clinic (Kendall),
Northwestern University (B. Riegel), and Princeton (E. Wallis),

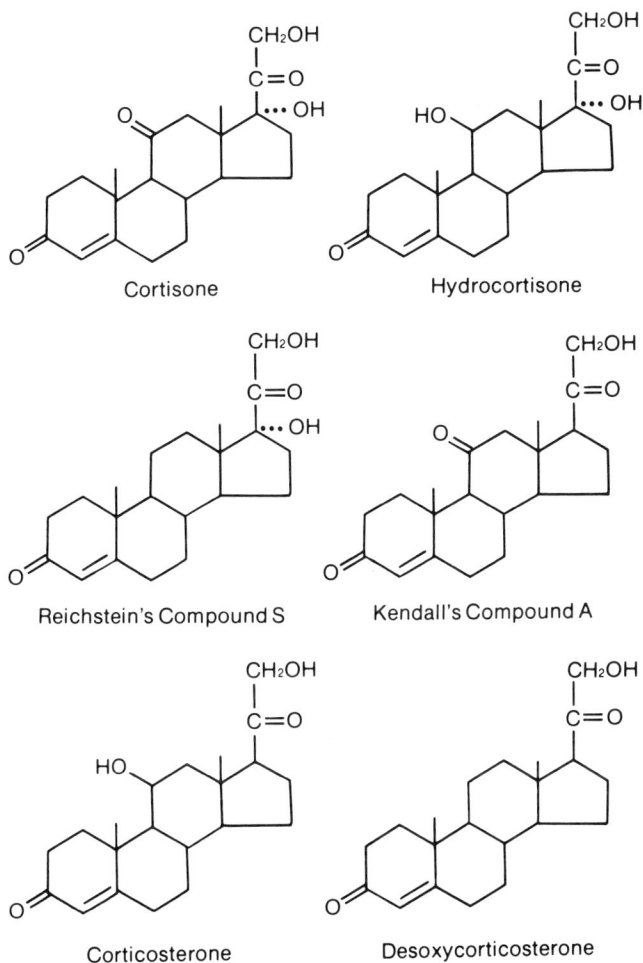

Cortisone

Hydrocortisone

Reichstein's Compound S

Kendall's Compound A

Corticosterone

Desoxycorticosterone

Figure 7. Major hormones of the human adrenal cortex.

and at the pharmaceutical firms Merck (L. H. Sarett) and
Squibb (O. Wintersteiner), attacked this problem. These groups
exchanged reports of their findings among themselves and with
Reichstein in Switzerland in order to move along as rapidly as
possible.

By 1946, principally through the efforts of Kendall and
Sarett, both Kendall's Compound A and cortisone had been
prepared on a small scale in the laboratory. Compound A,

which was easier to reach, was tested first and displayed no interesting activity in man. Despite their discouragement, the teams pressed on; by 1948 a large enough supply of cortisone had been prepared at Merck from ox bile to study its actions against human disease.

Cortisone

In May 1948, Sarett sent a sample of this cortisone to Kendall and Phillip Hench, a rheumatologist at Mayo. Hench had observed over the years that sufferers from rheumatoid arthritis often experienced remission (temporary cure) of their disease during pregnancy or when they fell ill with infectious jaundice. He believed that suppression of arthritic symptoms resulted from the action of steroid hormones released by the body in response to pregnancy or jaundice.

Hench reasoned that cortisone might have been the responsible hormone. In September 1948, be began to use Sarett's cortisone to treat a badly crippled female arthritic. Within a few days the patient experienced substantial relief of her symptoms. In particular, the swelling and inflammation of her tender joints subsided, so that she could move her limbs with freedom and resume physical activity. When the drug was withdrawn, the disease returned with all its former severity.

In April 1949, Hench and Kendall announced their discovery of the palliative actions of cortisone in rheumatic disease. The popular press extensively reported their findings, and arthritics all over the United States demanded the relief that the few at Mayo had experienced. The Merck firm responded to the demand with an all-out effort to mass produce cortisone. But it wasn't easy. The Sarett-Kendall process was the most complex organic chemical manufacturing system in existence up to that time. It employed a wide variety of techniques labeled as laboratory curiosities. By ingenuity and perseverance, Merck achieved commercial levels of production by late 1949. Schering (USA) followed with a similar process in 1951; other producers later entered the field. For a time fears arose that there was not enough ox bile in the world to supply the needs for cortisone manufacture. But with the persistent development efforts of steroid chemists in the pharmaceutical industry, production yields improved dramatically. As a result, the price of cortisone fell from $200 per gram in 1949 to $3.50 per gram in 1955.

As cortisone and later (1952) hydrocortisone, a closely related adrenocorticoid, were studied widely in medicine, many new and startling findings surfaced about the multifarious biological actions of this class of medicines. On the positive side of the ledger, a wide variety of serious dermatologic, allergic and collagen ailments yielded to their use. Eye and skin inflammations were often dramatically cured. The course of fatal diseases like nephrosis, pemphigus and lupus erythematosus could be stayed for long periods of time. Previously intractable asthma and hay fever responded promptly. Eventually these adrenocorticoids were found to be useful in treating more than 150 diseases.

Unfortunately, these drugs were not an unmixed blessing. While administration of moderate doses for short periods (several weeks or a month) was safe, employment of large doses over long intervals was fraught with danger. Prominent among undesirable side effects was retention of water and salt by the patient causing a puffy edematous condition accompanied by an increased burden on the heart and elevation of blood pressure. Occasionally stomach ulcers flared, fatty pads developed on the face and between the shoulders and after very long treatment, bones sometimes fractured spontaneously from drug-induced loss of calcium.

Some of the above deficiencies already had become apparent in the early 50s, and several U.S. pharmaceutical firms began a diligent search for agents resembling the corticosteroids in their beneficial actions but free of some or all of their drawbacks.

Safer Synthetic Analogs

The first breakthrough was achieved at the Schering Corporation (USA) in 1954. Chemists and microbiologists, working together, modified the structures of cortisone and hydrocortisone with the aid of microbes to produce prednisone and prednisolone, respectively. (See Figure 8).

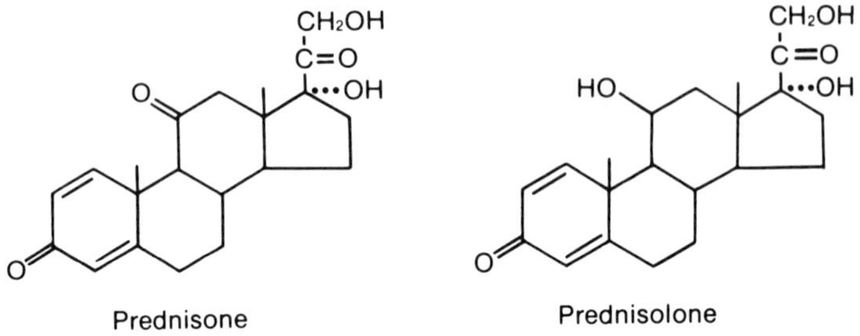

Figure 8. Improved, synthetic anti-inflammatory steroids.

In each case the chemical change involved the loss of two atoms of hydrogen from a structure containing 28 or 30 such atoms. Yet this minor alteration increased the potency of the resulting drugs three to five times over their parents and, best of all, abolished the salt-and-water-retaining side effect that had limited the use of cortisone and hydrocortisone. Schering introduced these medicines in 1955, following clinical evaluation at the National Institutes of Health, and they rapidly replaced cortisone and hydrocortisone for almost all indications.

With continued use, however, it became apparent that the other liabilities of corticosteroid therapy still applied to prednisone and prednisolone. Schering and other pharmaceutical firms (Merck, Upjohn, Lederle, Squibb) then brought forward a variety of modified corticosteroids derived from the prednisolone structure. Several of these were considerably more potent than prednisone and prednisolone, but none were free of dangers when taken by mouth or injection for prolonged periods. In recent years synthetic corticosteroids have come to be regarded as heroic therapy, to be used when all else fails. The exceptions to this trend have been their uses on skin and in eyes, where short-term treatments involving little or no absorption of the drug into the blood continue to benefit patients.

Polypeptides and Proteins

Finally, we turn to the classes of hormones, namely polypeptides and proteins, knowledge of which has been slowest to develop. Scientists recognized them in the earliest days of scientific hormone research. But few basic advances were achieved until the middle of the 20th century, because of the structural complexity of these agents and the lack of appropriate chemical tools to deal with them.

The importance of protein in living matter was first appreciated by the Dutch chemist Mulder as far back as 1838. At that time he introduced the term *protein*, derived from the Greek *prote* ("first") and *eidos* ("like"), to describe a material he had recognized to be common to many natural sources. Over the next 80 years, many of the giants of organic chemistry worked on the problem of protein structure. They separated these ubiquitous substances from widely diverse and even bizarre natural materials. Hemoglobin, the first protein to be crystallized, was obtained in 1840 by evaporating the blood of the earthworm. Globulin was isolated from the Brazil nut in 1877. Gradually an appreciation arose that the basic unit of the protein (and polypeptide) is the amino acid and that these units could be linked together in the laboratory through *peptide bond formation* to yield aggregates of higher molecular weight, which had some slight resemblance to the proteins from whence the amino acids were originally produced. (See Figure 9.)

However, the biological role of proteins as hormones (and their simpler, but closely related analogs, the polypeptides), distinct from that as the ground-substance for living matter, remained obscure.

The first systematic studies of a hormone, performed with the polypeptide secretin by Sir William Maddock Bayliss and Ernest Starling in 1904, as described at the beginning of this chapter, employed crude hormone preparations, the active content of which was only a tiny fraction of the total preparation. They had not, nor could they have had, any reasonable understanding of the composition of the active agent, since it had not been separated and purified. Even if these stages had been accomplished, detailed chemical identification would have been beyond the scope of the chemical science of that day.

Discovery of Insulin

Once the principle of hormone activity and function was established, important progress followed in the application of

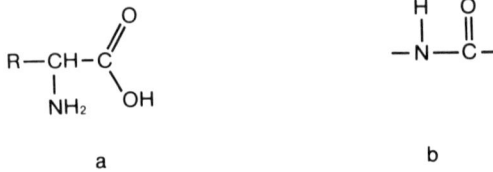

Figure 9. Structural units of polypeptides and proteins. a. A generic formula for alpha-amino acids, the basic structural unit of polypeptides and proteins. (R includes a variety of carbon, hydrogen, oxygen and nitrogen-containing alternatives.) b. The peptide bond, formed between the NH₂ group of one amino acid and the COOH group of another. The formation of these bonds is nature's way of fabricating polypeptides and proteins.

polypeptide hormones to medicine, in spite of a lack of basic chemical understanding. A striking example of this progress was the discovery of insulin. In 1869, Paul Langerhans described the islet cells, an element of structure of the pancreas. The function of these islets of Langerhans remained a mystery for about 20 years, after which the idea arose (from the work of many physiologists) that the health and function of these cells were somehow intimately related to the prevention of diabetes.

Following the work of G. R. Murray with thyroxine, and Bayliss and Starling with secretin, researchers attempted to prepare an extract of animal pancreas that could be used in treating diabetes. But either through lack of activity or because of toxicity, these extracts failed to produce the desired results.

In 1920, Frederick Banting, a Canadian orthopedic surgeon, conceived the idea that past failures to achieve a useful pancreatic extract were caused by the actions of impurities arising from sites in the pancreas other than the islets of Langerhans. Using methods already established by other physiologists for producing an atrophic dog pancreas composed substantially of islet cells, Banting and his co-worker, medical student Charles Best, prepared a pancreatic extract that was safe and effective for the treatment of experimental diabetes (the always necessary biological model). Recognizing the importance of their discovery, they then sought and found a plentiful source of islet cell material in the pancreas of the foetal calf, in which the remainder of the gland is substantially undeveloped. From these readily available organs, they prepared an extract that they injected first into themselves, to prove safety, and then into human diabetics.

The effects of these new extracts (called isletin first, and later insulin) on human diabetics were rapid and lifesaving. Elevated blood glucose levels returned to normal, and debilitating signs of the disease disappeared. With the development of carefully standardized insulin preparations, the diabetic could, by balancing the carbohydrate and carbohydrate-generating elements of his diet against his need for insulin supplement, lead a reasonably normal life. For his contribution to this remarkable advance in hormone therapy, Banting received the Nobel Prize with McLeod, in whose laboratory the work was done. Banting publicly acknowledged Best's role in the discovery by sharing the award with him.

In 1926, insulin was isolated as a pure, crystalline substance by J. J. Abel (mentioned earlier for his work with epinephrine), and was in time shown indisputably to belong to the polypeptide class. However, progress in the application of other protein and polypeptide hormones to the treatment of disease continued to be very slow.

ACTH

In 1946, on the initiative of the Armour Co., a large meat packer, a polypeptide hormone of the pituitary called the adrenocorticotrophic hormone (ACTH) was made available to the medical profession. This extract of porcine pituitary could stimulate the adrenal to produce hydrocortisone and other normal products of adrenal cortex activity. Consequently, ACTH was later applied to the treatment of conditions that also responded to the administration of cortisone or hydrocortisone. Unfortunately, in common with other polypeptide and protein hormones, it had to be injected, while cortisone could be given by mouth. This has inhibited major use of ACTH, even though it has the advantage of stimulating normal-type adrenal activity, whereas cortisone and other adrenocortical steroids suppress that activity.

Oxytocin

A second development of the late 40s, sponsored by the Detroit pharmaceutical firm Parke-Davis, was the introduction of another hormone of the pituitary called oxytocin. Intravenous administration of this hormone to women in late pregnancy brings on labor when it fails to start spontaneously.

During and after World War II, new tools of great power reinforced the techniques of chemistry. As a result, progress in all fields of organic chemistry, especially in the polypeptide field, escalated. Vincent Du Vigneaud and his group at Cornell University Medical School were able to crystallize a salt of oxytoxin in 1952 and, by 1954, had determined its structure as well as devised a laboratory method for its synthesis. For this breakthrough, the first complete description of a polypeptide hormone, Du Vigneaud received the Nobel Prize in 1955. Following Du Vigneaud's success, research workers elsewhere reported the structures and syntheses of insulin and of ACTH. Although, in contrast with other hormone classes, it often remains most convenient to use animal sources for the polypeptides and proteins, the simplest, oxytocin, is now manufactured synthetically by Sandoz, a Swiss pharmaceutical firm, and even the complex ACTH is synthesized by CIBA-GEIGY in Switzerland.

More recent study has dealt with modification and simplification of those complex hormone structures, an area of research presently recognized as the major task of hormone chemistry for the years ahead.

Suggested Reading

Applezweig, N. *Steroid Drugs.* (Vol. 1.) New York: Blakiston, Div. McGraw Hill, 1962.

Du Vigneaud, V. Trail of Sulfur Research: From Insulin to Oxytocin. *Science*, 1956, *123*, 967.

Maisal, A. A. *The Hormone Quest.* New York: Random House, 1965.

Pharmaceutical Manufacturers Association. Progress in Drug Research. (PMA Symposium) *Bulletin*, 1969, *69*-(3).

Sexton, W. A. *Chemical Constitution and Biological Activity.* (3rd ed.) Princeton: Van Nostrand, 1963.

Singer, D., & Underwood, A. E. *Short History of Medicine.* (2nd ed.) New York: Oxford University Press, 1962.

CHAPTER 7

Chemical Transmitters and the Control of Blood Pressure

Albert J. Plummer
George deStevens

Nearly 18 million Americans suffer from hypertension (high blood pressure). Complications commonly due to this insidious disease—arteriosclerosis, kidney disease, cerebral hemorrhage and coronary artery disease—cause more than half of the adult deaths each year in the United States.

As recently as 25 years ago, the prevailing medical view was that elevated blood pressure was a protective compensatory adjustment to an ill-defined increase in the circulatory demands of the individual. Many even believed that lowering of the pressure would be harmful.

Until 1949 no effective drugs existed for controlling hypertension. But in a span of only 20 years since then, successive research gains have clearly shown that drug therapy can reduce blood pressure to normal range, much to the advantage—rather than detriment—of the patient.

The first known measurement of blood pressure was carried out in a horse in 1732 by Stephen Hales, an English clergyman. Hales measured the blood pressure by inserting a brass pipe tightly fitted to a nine foot vertical glass tube into an artery of the neck. This method, which presented many serious problems, was of course not applicable to man. In fact, nearly two centuries elapsed before the Russian physician N. S. Korotov, developed the simple, safe and reliable pressure cuff technique now used everywhere.

The systolic blood pressure (crest of pressure wave) of a healthy young man, taken when sitting, reads 120 mm. Hg (mercury) with a range of 90 to 120 mm.; his diastolic pressure (trough of pressure wave) records 80 mm. with a range of 60 to 80 mm. In hypertension, however, it is not uncommon to find systolic and diastolic pressures of double the normal values. In carefully controlled studies of a large group of people over several decades in Framingham, Massachusetts, the risk of heart attack appeared to be four times greater for a person with a systolic blood pressure of 160 mm. Hg than for one with a pressure of 120 mm.

Sympathetic Nervous System

It has long been known that stimulation of a sympathetic nerve causes constriction of the small arteries (arterioles) in the region affected by the nerve. The sympathetic nervous system also regulates the degree of constriction of the arterioles so as to keep blood pressure from fluctuating excessively upon changing position (for example, from lying to standing or the reverse). Partial constriction maintains a normal blood pressure; if the influence of the sympathetic nerves on the blood vessels vanished, the blood pressure would drop excessively, because the volume of the vascular space would far exceed that of the contained blood.

Discovery of Neurotransmitters

In 1920, Otto Loewi first demonstrated in the frog that stimulation of the sympathetic nerves causes the release of a chemical substance. In his classic experiment, he isolated the hearts of two frogs—the first with its nerves, the second without them. Both hearts were attached to glass tubes and filled with Ringer's solution. When the sympathetic nerve was stimulated for a few minutes, and the Ringer's solution was transferred to the second heart, the second heart speeded. Thus, he demonstrated that sympathetic nerves do not influence the heart directly but, from their endings, release specific chemicals— neurotransmitters—that in turn bring about the observed effect. In the frog the neurotransmitter was epinephrine; in man it was found to be norepinephrine.

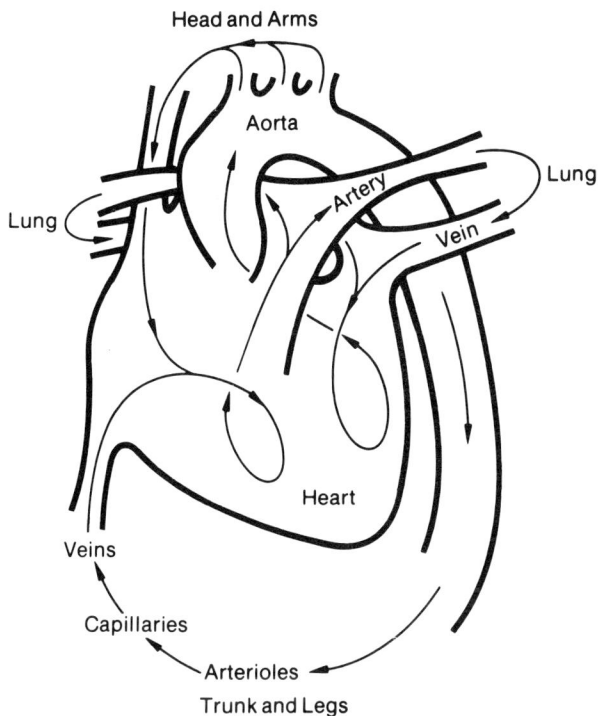

Figure 1. Diagram of circulation. Dark, bluish-red blood in the veins returns from the body and is pumped to the lungs where it picks up a fresh supply of oxygen and becomes bright red. It returns to the heart and is pumped via the aorta to the arteries to be distributed again in the body.

Adrenergic Blocking Agent

Loewi also demonstrated that ergotamine prevented the speeding of the second frog heart but did not prevent release of the epinephrine-like substance by stimulation of the sympathetic nerve to the first heart. Ergotamine was designated as an adrenergic blocking agent, a name given to compounds that can block the blood pressure rise caused by stimulation of the sympathetic nerves supplying the heart and blood vessels.

Catecholamines

In 1946, U. S. von Euler of the Karolinska Institute in Stockholm established that in mammals, including man, the sympathetic neurotransmitter is norepinephrine rather than the epinephrine found in the frog. Epinephrine (adrenaline) is the major neurohumor in the adrenal medulla in man, but norepinephrine is localized at the nerve endings. Epinephrine and norepinephrine are closely related catecholamines with the chemical structures illustrated below.

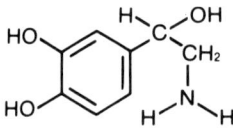

Norepinephrine   Epinephrine

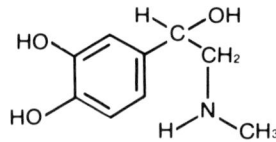

Sympathectomy

By about 1940, neurosurgeons had shown that removal of portions of the sympathetic nervous system from the chest and abdomen, a procedure known as a sympathectomy, lowers the blood pressure in hypertension by reducing the resistance of the arterioles toward the normal range. In time this surgical procedure prompted many investigators to search for ways to achieve the same results by means of a chemical sympathectomy—that is, through the use of drugs.

Sympathetic Nervous Pathway

The highest centers of the sympathetic nervous system (See Figure 2) lie in the hypothalamic area of the midbrain. From these centers, nervous pathways pass down the spinal cord and out into the ganglia at both sides of the vertebrae in the chest and abdomen. The ganglia on each side of the spinal cord are connected in a long chain that extends through the chest and abdomen. Within each ganglion a synapse (space) separates the preganglionic from the postganglionic nerve.

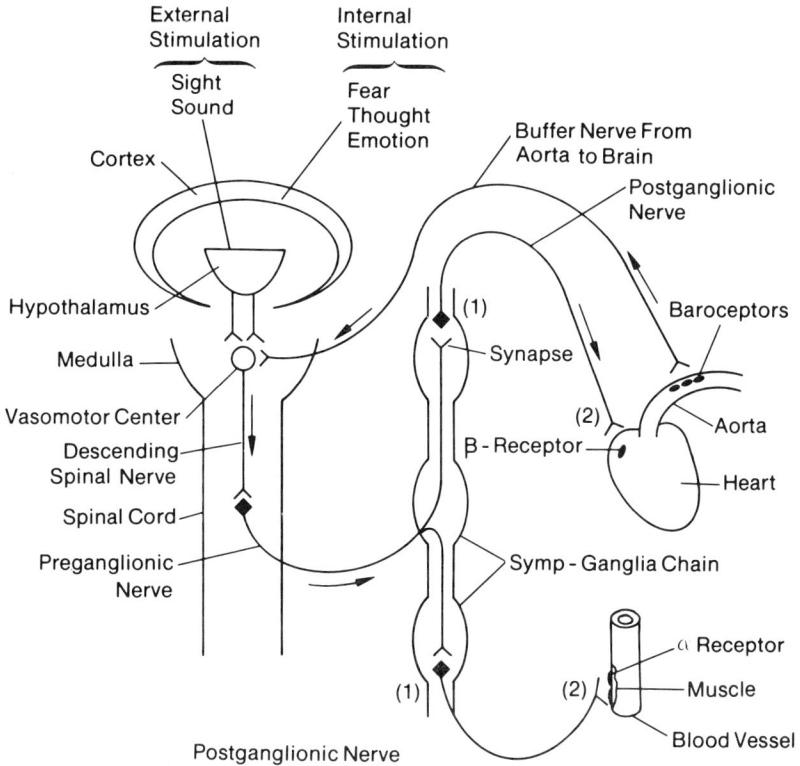

Figure 2. Schematic diagram of the sympathetic nervous system. Acetylcholine is liberated at (1). Norepinephrine is liberated at (2).

An impulse coming along a preganglionic nerve crosses over the synapse to the postganglionic nerve by means of a chemical mediator (humor). This process is called a neurohumoral transmission. (See Figure 3.) In this case the neurohumor is acetylcholine. When an impulse reaches the nerve ending it releases the acetylcholine, which carries the impulse across the synapse to the postganglionic nerve.

Fibers from the postganglionic nerve ending pass to the receptor of the arteriolar muscle. The neurohumor norepinephrine is stored in granules at the postganglionic nerve ending. When the impulse reaches the postganglionic nerve ending, it releases the

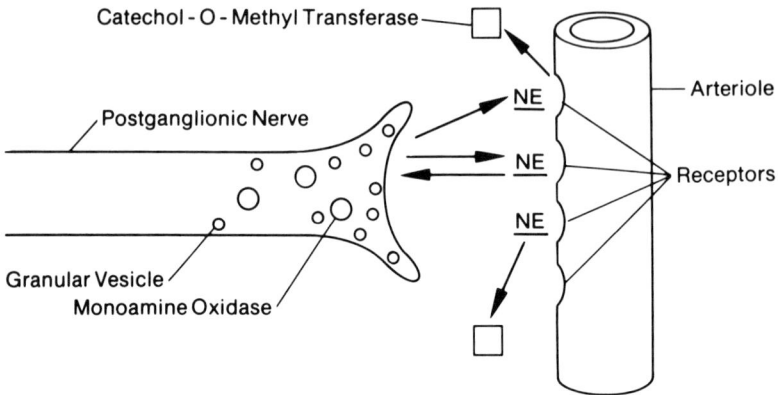

Figure 3. Schematic diagram of neurohumoral transmission. Nor-epinephrine (NE) liberated from granular vesicles by nerve impulses passes through cell membrane to reach receptors, causing activation and muscle contraction. Norepinephrine passes back into nerve fibers and is taken up by vesicles again or destroyed by monoamine oxidase; some diffuses away and is inactivated by catechol-O-methyl trans-ferase. Reserpine liberates norepinephrine from granules and also blocks entry of dopamine into granules where it is converted to norepinephrine.

norepinephrine, which crosses over to the receptor. The nor-epinephrine-receptor interaction triggers contraction of the arteriolar muscle and narrows the arteriole, thus causing a rise in blood pressure.

The action ends when the norepinephrine passes back into the storage granule of the nerve fiber. (See Figure 3.) Two enzymes destroy excess norepinephrine: (a) monoamine oxidase within the nerve cell, and (b) catechol-O-methyltransferase, which is extracellular.

Electrical stimulation of an animal's sympathetic centers activates its entire sympathetic system and releases norepine-phrine at widespread vascular sites, producing a rise in blood pressure. In similar fashion, fear, tension, apprehension, excite-ment and anxiety—emotional states that arise in higher centers of the brain at the level of the cortex—may act on the sympa-thetic center to initiate sympathetic nerve impulses that con-strict the arterioles and increase blood pressure. The nervous pathways from the cortex to the sympathetic centers are not precisely defined, but man can elevate his blood pressure merely by thought alone.

A drug may exert a suppressant effect at several points along the sympathetic nervous pathway: (a) sympathetic centers within the midbrain, (b) junction within a sympathetic ganglion and (c) junction between the nerve and the blood vessel. Other less well-defined areas of the brain also may be involved, and, finally, responsiveness of the arteriolar muscle to the neurohumor may be reduced.

Parasympathetic Nervous System

The parasympathetic nervous system has a center in the brain close to the sympathetic center and regulates the same organs— but in reverse fashion. For example, parasympathetic activity causes dilation of the blood vessels of the abdominal viscera, as well as cardiac slowing, decrease in size of pupil and increased flow of saliva—quite the opposite of the effects of the sympathetic system. In this system, acetylcholine is the neurohumor liberated at both the ganglia and the postganglionic nerve endings.

Baroceptors

In everyday life, blood pressure is read by pressure-sensitive baroceptors in the arch of the aorta, in the right auricle of the heart, and at junctions of the carotid arteries in the neck. The baroceptors send nervous impulses to the sympathetic centers. (See Figure 4.)

A rise in blood pressure increases the frequency of impulse reaching the sympathetic centers. The centers respond to this braking action, as it were, by reducing the frequency of nerve impulses to the blood vessels, thus relaxing the arteriolar muscle and lowering the elevated pressure. A drop in blood pressure decreases the frequency of impulses reaching the sympathetic center and causes a compensatory rise in pressure. This delicately balanced mechanism curbs the excessive drop in blood pressure commonly associated with dizziness.

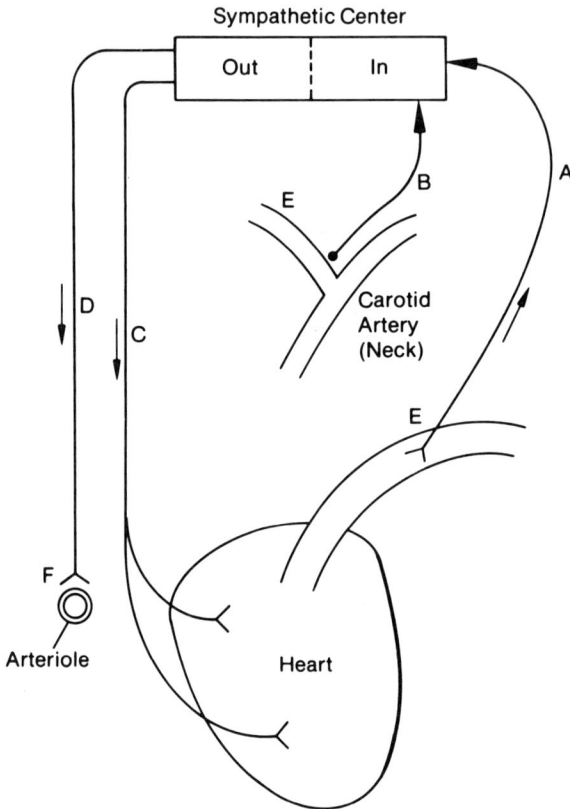

Figure 4. Schematic diagram of sympathetic/baroceptor system. Nerve impulses originate in the pressure sensitive centers (E). A fall in pressure in the aorta or the carotid artery results in transmission of nerve impulses via the ascending nerves A or B to the sympathetic center. A compensating impulse then travels via the descending sympathetic nerves C and D and leads to a relaxation of the arteriole F, slowing of the heart rate, and a reduction in cardiac force (output) with a resultant fall in blood pressure.

Alpha and Beta Receptors

Early investigators of the sympathetic nervous system were puzzled when they observed that epinephrine injected in very low concentrations caused a drop in blood pressure, while at moderate or higher dosage the blood pressure rose. R. P.

Ahlquist explained this paradox by suggesting that there are not one but two types of sympathetic receptors—the alpha and the beta types. This concept, now well accepted, is based on the different effects of three catecholamines—epinephrine, norepinephrine and isopropylnorepinephrine (isoproterenol)—on the receptors.

Isopropylnorepinephrine (isoproterenol) is not made by the animal body but is a synthetic compound that is a valuable tool for stimulating beta receptors.

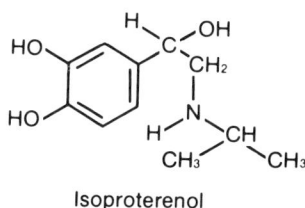

Isoproterenol

Action of the catecholamines on the receptors is as follows:

	Alpha receptors	Beta receptors
Epinephrine	marked	moderate
Norepinephrine	moderate	weak
Isoproterenol	weak	marked

The current view is that these receptors have a molecular configuration for which the neurohumor has an affinity by virtue of its size and shape and that their interaction detonates a response in the receptor which causes the cell to react. According to this concept, a blocker (alpha or beta) has an affinity for the receptor, but their interaction does not activate the receptor. The blocker is so bound that it impedes access of the neurohumor to the receptor, thus blocking the response of the muscle.

Neurohumoral stimulation (See Figure 5) of the beta receptors (which are most abundant in arteriolar muscles of the skeletal system) leads to relaxation of the arteriolar muscle and dilation of the blood vessels. Stimulation of the alpha receptors

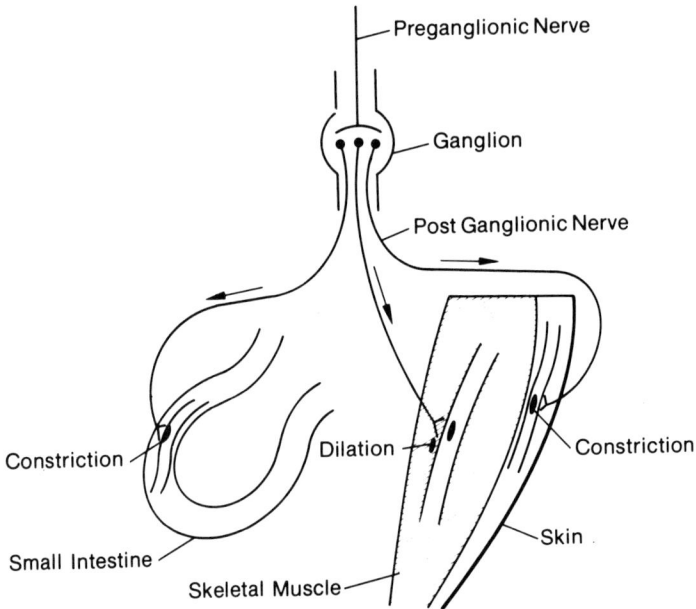

Figure 5. Sketch of sympathetic vascular receptors. Sympathetic nerve impulses release neurohumor which acts on alpha receptors to constrict blood vessels of small intestine and skin and upon beta receptors to relax blood vessels of skeletal muscle.

(which predominate in the skin and the abdominal viscera) causes a contraction of the arteriolar muscle and a narrowing of the blood vessels. The result of these opposing influences is the algebraic sum of alpha- and beta-mediated actions, that is, a rise in blood pressure following use of epinephrine or norepinephrine and a drop in blood pressure following use of isoproterenol.

Alpha and Beta Blocking Agents

An alpha-adrenergic blocking agent binds to the alpha receptor and permits epinephrine to bind only to the beta receptor. The unopposed dilation of the blood vessels results in a fall in blood pressure, rather than the usual blood pressure increase. This unmasks a relaxation of blood vessels and hypotensive effect which is normally overshadowed by the more marked constrictor effect. This phenomenon, employed in the laboratory to uncover alpha adrenergic blocking compounds, is called epinephrine reversal.

All three amines—with isoproterenol being most effective—increase the rate and force of the heart through stimulation of the beta receptors. By the same token, rate and force of the heart are reduced by application of a beta-adrenergic blocking agent which prevents the stimulatory action of all three amines. Propanolol is typical of the class of beta-adrenergic blocking agents. Its structural formula closely resembles that of isoproterenol, the beta receptor stimulant. The obvious similarity in the shapes of their molecules allows the two compounds to bind with the same beta receptor.

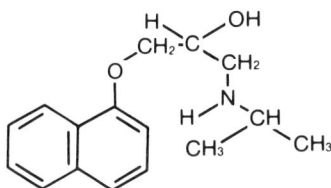

Propranolol

Unlike the arrangement in the arterioles, there are no clearly defined alpha receptors that exert an effect opposite to that of the beta receptor on cardiac action. This function is under control of the parasympathetic or vagus nerve to the heart. Acetylcholine, the neurohumor liberated by stimulation of the vagus nerve, reacts with parasympathetic receptors to slow the rate and reduce the force of the heart.

Antihypertensive Mechanisms

Alpha-Adrenergic Blockade

The first compounds to receive serious consideration as antihypertensive drugs were the alpha-adrenergic blocking agents. They do not interfere with liberation of norepinephrine from the synergistic nerves close to the blood vessels but prevent any action by occupying the binding sites of the alpha receptors.

Phentolamine and piperoxan are examples of adrenergic blockers studied in the late 40s, but the hope that they might be beneficial in human hypertension evaporated. Although alpha adrenergic blockade achieved a concurrent drop in blood pressure, the heart rate markedly accelerated because the beta receptors were not blocked and, in fact, were stimulated by the sympathetic neurohumor liberated near the heart pacemaker in response to the drop in blood pressure. This action was initiated by activation of the baroceptors in the aorta and carotid arteries in response to the drop in arterial pressure. The consequent rapid heart rate and increased cardiac force gave rise to unpleasant subjective feelings in the chest and tended to combat any possible hypotensive effect.

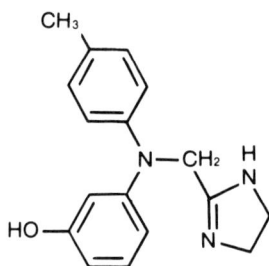

Phentolamine

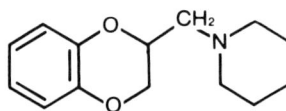

Piperoxan

The alpha blockers, however, found a very important clinical application in diagnosis of pheochromocytoma, an adrenal tumor. This tumor secretes excessive amounts of catecholamines into the circulation. The high blood pressure that follows promptly falls when adrenergic blockers are injected intravenously. In contrast, essential hypertension resists these compounds. It is thus possible to diagnose the presence of this type of tumor. Such blocking agents also make it possible to protect patients against the deleterious effects of excess catecholamines, which are expressed into the circulation during surgical removal of the tumor.

Ganglionic Blockade

The availability of potent ganglionic blocking agents that suppress the action of acetylcholine at the ganglionic synapse of the sympathetic nerve led to development of the first effective medicines for treatment of hypertension.

Since 1899, nicotine had been known to block the sympathetic nervous pathways at the ganglionic synapse, but no therapeutic advantage ensued because of nicotine's high toxicity. The first compound of this type to show therapeutic value, hexamethonium, was investigated by W. D. M. Paton and Eleanor Zaimis in England in 1948. Hexamethonium is a bisquaternary compound with two trimethylammonium centers separated by six methylene groups. Comparison of **its** formula with that of acetylcholine shows an obvious similarity that explains the competition of the two compounds for the same receptor site.

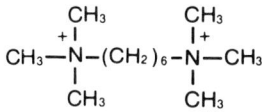

$$CH_3-\overset{\overset{\displaystyle CH_3}{+|}}{N}-(CH_2)_6-\overset{\overset{\displaystyle CH_3}{|+}}{N}-CH_3$$
$$||$$
$$CH_3CH_3$$

Hexamethonium

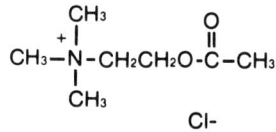

$$CH_3-\overset{\overset{\displaystyle CH_3}{+|}}{N}-CH_2CH_2O-\overset{\overset{\displaystyle O}{||}}{C}-CH_3$$
$$|$$
$$CH_3 \qquad Cl-$$

Acetylocholine

Sympathetic pathways to both alpha and beta receptors are interrupted at the ganglia. Ganglionic blockade thus provides an advantage over the alpha adrenergic blockers in that no undesirable speeding of the heart accompanies the drop in blood pressure. However, poor oral absorption hampers the effectiveness of hexamethonium. The more readily absorbed compounds chlorisondamine and mecamylamine largely overcame this problem. The latter is unusual in that it is not a quaternary salt and thus constituted a departure from the presumed structural requirements of ganglionic blockers.

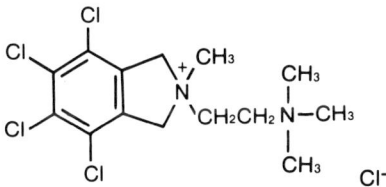

Chlorisondamine Chloride

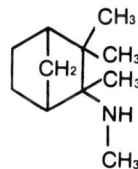

Mecamylamine

The main disadvantages of such compounds result from the blockade of both sympathetic and parasympathetic ganglia, with consequent dryness of the mouth, visual disturbance and constipation. Still, they provided for the first time conclusive evidence that a substance that lowered blood pressure in normotensive laboratory animals could also be effective in human hypertension.

Direct Relaxation of Arterioles

The next drug to assume importance as an effective antihypertensive agent emerged on the therapeutic scene in 1952. It was hydralazine, prepared by Jean Druey of CIBA-Basle.

In animals hydralazine causes a drop in blood pressure that is more gradual and more prolonged than that produced by the ganglionic blockers. Another advantage is that an increase in dosage leads to an increase in duration rather than in magnitude of the blood pressure drop. Hydralazine also elevates blood flow to the kidney. Since decreased blood flow contributes to renal hypertension, this action is desirable.

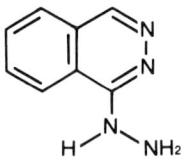

Hydralazine

Relaxation of the arterioles brings about the hydralazine-induced drop in blood pressure. This effect accelerates the heart by activating the baroceptors and sympathetic nerves to the beta receptors of the heart, as described earlier for the alpha adrenergic blockers. Hydralazine is not, however, an alpha adrenergic blocker in therapeutic doses. It decreases the blood pressure rise caused by administration of norepinephrine, but it also suppresses the constrictor effect of barium chloride and angiotensin, two agents that act directly on the arteriolar muscle. It therefore appears that hydralazine definitely acts on the muscle itself rather than on its sympathetic nerve supply.

Henry Schroeder, in St. Louis in 1954, succeeded in preventing the cardiac speeding encountered in hypertensive patients treated with hydralazine by combining it with the ganglionic blocking agent, hexamethonium. This new approach dampened the sympathetic nervous action responsible for the rapid heart rate. Another advantage of such combination therapy is that it enables the dose, and hence the side effects, of each individual drug to be reduced. It is noteworthy that dihydralazine, the dihydrazino derivative of phthalazine, has been used outside the United States as an antihypertensive for well over a decade. Its mechanism of action appears to be the same as that of hydralazine.

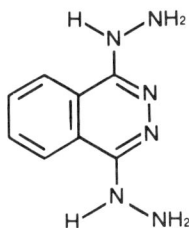

Dihydralazine

Depletion of Sympathetic Neurohumor

Reserpine, an alkaloid obtained from an Indian plant, Rauwolfia serpentina, joined the group of useful antihypertensive drugs less than two years after the appearance of hydralazine. It differs from the earlier drugs in that it provides quieting and sedation in addition to its subtle hypotensive action. This substance was extracted from the Rauwolfia plant by Johannes Müller and Emil Schlittler of CIBA-Basle in 1952.

The central nervous and circulatory effects of reserpine, first noted by Professor Hugo Bein, also of CIBA-Basle, came on gradually and persisted for several days in animals after a single oral dose. Surprisingly, the drop in blood pressure was associated with a slowing of the heart rate rather than the customary reflex speeding. This suggested that the activity of the entire sympathetic nervous system, including the beta receptors, had been reduced. This proved to be the case; in 1955 M. Holzbauer

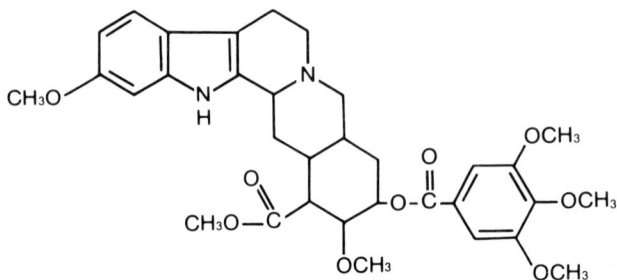

Reserpine

and Marthe Vogt in England and Arvid Carlsson and N. A. Hillarp in Sweden learned independently that reserpine frees norepinephrine from its binding sites in the granules both in the central sympathetic centers and in the sympathetic nerve terminals that impinge on the arterioles. The released norepinephrine is destroyed by monoamine oxidase. It followed logically that the arteriolar relaxation, cardiac slowing and drop in blood pressure stemmed from depletion of the neurohumor on which the function of the sympathetic nervous system depends. This is a chemical sympathectomy in the strictest sense of the word. The quieting action of reserpine is also important, especially in human hypertension, since sedation can be beneficial where anxiety contributes to the hypertension. The hypotensive effects of reserpine observed in animals—gradual onset and long duration—were fully duplicated in human medicine where the drug has found wide application.

Reserpine not only liberates norepinephrine from its storage site in the granular vesicles of the sympathetic nerves to permit its destruction by monoamine oxidase, but the drug also interferes with the synthesis of norepinephrine by preventing entry of the precursor, dopamine, into the granules. Normally dopamine is hydroxylated in the granule to form norepinephrine.

This brief description of the action of reserpine represents intensive efforts by many workers over the past 15 years. The area remains under active study.

In addition to its efficacy as a medicine, reserpine has become a valuable tool for pharmacologists. By releasing the catecholamines of the sympathetic nervous system from their binding sites, reserpine has provided insights into the finer details of the biochemical processes responsible for the function of the system. Not since J. N. Langley in the last century first mapped the sympathetic ganglia through the use of nicotine has so much significant new information been obtained through the aid of a single chemical.

In 1959 Robert Mull at CIBA prepared a compound of a novel chemical structure and Robert Maxwell and Albert Plummer evaluated it biologically. This substance, a guanidyl derivative containing an eight-member ring known as guanethidine marked a significant advance in the treatment of hypertension. As with reserpine, it acts primarily on the peripheral sympathetic nerves where it initially depletes the neurohumor from its storage site. The first phase is superseded by a persistent state during which the release of norepinephrine by nerve impulses arriving at the nerve terminals is impeded. The latter effect, important for its hypotensive action, is due to an interference with the passage of norepinephrine back into the nerve cell after release and to an inhibition of the uptake of norepinephrine by the storage granule within the nerve cell ending. Reserpine shares the action on the storage mechanism but does not interfere with the return of released norepinephrine into the nerve cell.

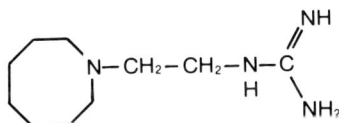

• ½ H_2SO_4

Guanethidine

Later studies revealed that guanethidine actually accumulates in the storage granules in the sympathetic terminals and occupies the site normally filled by norepinephrine. The affinity for this binding site is undoubtedly a factor in the displacement of norepinephrine from the storage granule. Because of the interference with the release of the sympathetic neurohumor there ensues a relaxation of the blood vessels, a fall in heart rate and a drop in blood pressure both in laboratory animals and in hypertensive patients. The effect of a single effective dose of guanethidine to an animal develops gradually over six hours and usually persists for 10 to 14 days. This sustained effect helps to regulate human hypertension smoothly.

Guanethidine does not act significantly at the ganglia, so it does not cause the dry mouth or visual disturbance experienced after ganglionic blockade. Its action on the sympathetic nerves resembles that of reserpine, but it fails to induce sedation, since it does not pass the barrier between the blood and the brain. Thus, guanethidine can bring about an even more selective chemical sympathectomy than reserpine, since its action is directed at the sympathetic nerve transmission from nerves to heart and blood vessels to the exclusion of any effect on the higher centers.

Since 1960, several guanidine-type compounds have been prepared in a number of laboratories and have been studied clinically. The following have exhibited antihypertensive activity:

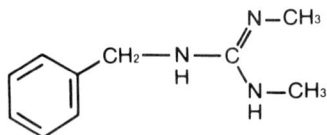

Bethanidine

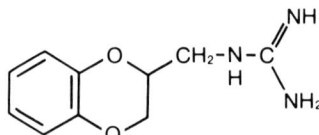

Guanoxan

Interference with Norepinephrine Synthesis

With realization that reserpine lowers blood pressure by reducing the availability of norepinephrine at sympathetic nerve endings, scientists sought to duplicate the effect by blocking the synthesis through enzymatic inhibition. Norepinephrine is derived from tyrosine, an essential amino acid in protein, in a series of three enzymatic steps illustrated below.

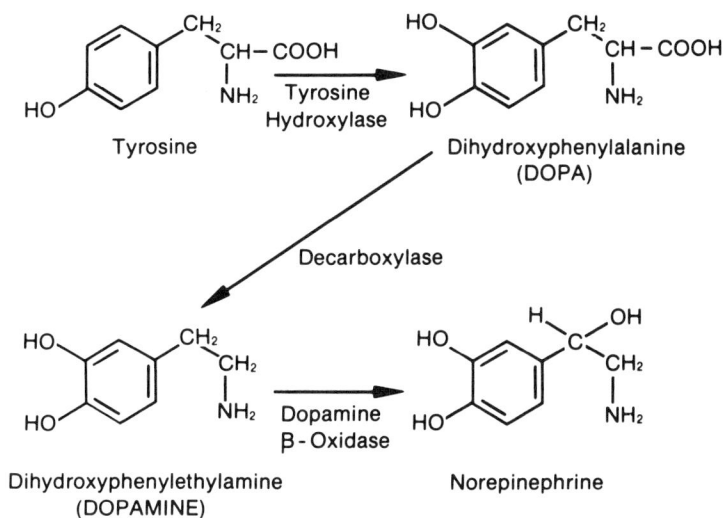

Theodore Sourkes, in 1954, discovered alphamethyldopa, the first effective inhibitor of the synthesis of norepinephrine. This substance blocked the decarboxylation in the second step of the synthesis. It did not appear to lower blood pressure in laboratory animals, and it was not until 1960 that John Oates noted its antihypertensive action in man via studies on amino acid metabolism. Like reserpine and unlike guanethidine, it has a sedative effect. The hypotensive mechanism is not precisely understood. It depletes norepinephrine from sympathetic nerves, but fails to reduce their activity. Significantly, alpha-methylmetatyrosine, another decarboxylase inhibitor closely related in structure to alphamethyldopa, even more effectively depletes norepinephrine from the nerves. But it does not lower blood pressure. This contrasts to experiences after guanethidine and reserpine, where the depression of sympathetic nerve function is better correlated with the degree of depletion of norepinephrine.

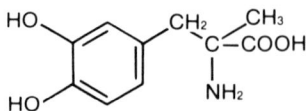

Alphamethyldopa

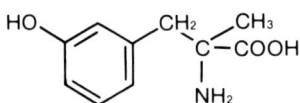

Alphamethylmetatyrosine   Alphamethylparatyrosine

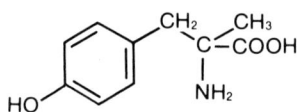

We know that alphamethyldopa converts to alphamethylnor-epinephrine. On this basis a "false transmitter" theory suggests that alphamethylnorepinephrine usurps the position of nor-epinephrine at the nerve ending and acts as its substitute. Although this may be so, it does not satisfactorily explain the reduced effect on the blood vessels, since alphamethylnor-epinephrine has a constrictor effect close to that of nor-epinephrine.

In 1965, Sidney Spector showed that another substance, alphamethylparatyrosine, blocks the synthesis of norepine-phrine at the first step by preventing the hydroxylation of tyrosine. The structure of this inhibitor is strikingly similar to the carboxylase inhibitors, alphamethyldopa and alphamethyl-metatyrosine. Although alphamethylparatyrosine can reduce norepinephrine to very low levels in sympathetic nerves, it does not significantly lower blood pressure in laboratory animals. It appears that depletion of the gross stores of the neurohumor in sympathetic nerves, by interfering with its synthesis, does not necessarily lead to a depression of sympathetic nervous activity. There is probably a smaller pool of norepinephrine, which is important for the function of the nerves, and this pool must be affected to dampen sympathetic nervous activity.

In any case, a precise explanation for the mechanism of the antihypertensive action of alphamethyldopa in man must await further study. The most recent evidence suggests that its actual locus of action may be on the central sympathetic centers.

Monoamine Oxidase Inhibition

Monoamine oxidase is an enzyme present in the mitochondria of sympathetic nerve endings. It functions there to neutralize excess norepinephrine by oxidation and removal of its amino group. Inhibition of the enzyme should increase rather than decrease the norepinephrine content of sympathetic nerves. Reserpine and guanethidine produce an opposite effect. Yet the study of the monoamine oxidase inhibitors in correcting mental depression (See Chapter 5) noted that they caused a drop in blood pressure, which has led to clinical use of the enzyme inhibitor pargyline for treating hypertension. The action here appears to be based on a reduction of arteriolar peripheral resistance, but despite much study the mechanism by which the resistance is lowered remains unknown. An important consideration in the use of an agent of this type is that many commonly used drugs, such as antihistamines, are amines whose action is normally terminated through deamination by monoamine oxidase. An inhibitor, therefore, prolongs the action of many potent medicines to the point of toxic manifestations and exaggerated effects. Certain cheeses, wines and beers contain tyramine, an amine that raises blood pressure. Severe hypertensive episodes can occur when patients inadvertently consume them while being treated with a monoamine oxidase inhibitor.

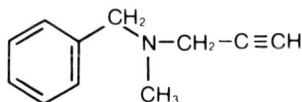

$$\text{C}_6\text{H}_5-\text{CH}_2-\overset{\underset{|}{\text{CH}_3}}{\text{N}}-\text{CH}_2-\text{C}\equiv\text{CH}$$

Pargyline

Antihypertensive Action of Diuretics

Diuretics increase the excretion of sodium chloride and water in the urine. Organic mercurial compounds had, for many years,

been the mainstays for this purpose, but in 1957 two nonmer-
curial sulfonamides, chlorothiazide and hydrochlorothiazide,
drastically altered diuretic therapy. (The discovery of the
thiazides has been described in Chapter 4.)

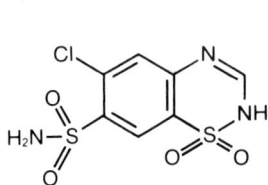

Chlorothiazide   Hydrochlorothiazide

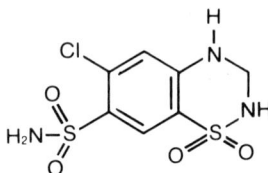

   James Sprague and Frederick Novello prepared chlorothiazide
at Merck Laboratories and George deStevens and Lincoln
Werner of CIBA Laboratories synthesized hydrochlorothiazide.
In independent clinical studies, Robert Wilkins in Boston and
Edward Freis in Washington noted that these substances cause a
moderate but definite lowering of the blood pressure in human
hypertension but do not alter normal blood pressure. These
diuretics have no noteworthy influence on normal blood pressure in laboratory animals but do lower elevated blood pressure
induced by a variety of experimental procedures. It is generally
though not universally deduced that the hypotensive effect of
diuretics is related to their diuretic action. Hence a reduction of
the water and sodium chloride content of the walls of the
arterioles in turn reduces the responsivity of the arterioles to
constrictor influences. In this connection A. Grollman had
shown earlier that a low salt diet tends to lower high blood
pressure in humans.

   It is especially significant in this regard that the constrictor
effects on arterioles of the sympathetic neurohumors, epinephrine and norepinephrine, were suppressed by hydrochlorothiazide pretreatment in dogs. Therefore, the most likely
cause of the antihypertensive action of these thiazides is a
decrease in vascular responsiveness to sympathetic amines,
whatever may be the underlying mechanism.

   Hydrochlorothiazide pre-treatment increases the drop in
blood pressure produced by hydralazine in the normotensive

dog, even though the blood pressure is not lowered by the diuretic itself. Since this inital observation, scientists have shown that the thiazide diuretics enhance the antihypertensive action of many medicines, including the ganglionic blockers, reserpine, syrosingopine and guanethidine. Such combinations have the advantage of smaller doses for an equivalent effect, with a consequent lessening of the side effects of each substance.

Summary

Major control of the level of arterial blood pressure is exerted through the sympathetic nervous system, which performs this function by neurohumoral regulation of the resistance to the flow of blood from the heart through the small arterioles and by its influence, on the function of the heart itself. Although sympathetic nervous overactivity has never been definitely implicated in the genesis of the overcontracted arteriolar state found in essential hypertension, it stays high on many investigators' lists of suspects as a distinct possibility. From the standpoint of treating hypertension, the sympathetic nervous system has served as the prime target of attack for drugs designed to correct the aberration.

Practically every effective antihypertensive agent has been shown to act as a barrier to the transit of sympathetic nervous impulses by reducing the availability of norepinephrine at some point between the brain and the arteriolar muscle. In the few types of antihypertensive drugs whose exact site of action has not been conclusively established, strong presumptive evidence suggests an involvement with the neurohumoral action of the sympathetic nervous system.

In a few short years, scientific advances have transformed the therapeutic management of essential hypertension from one of gross empiricism and dubious benefit to that of an orderly rational approach based on sound pharmacological principles. This progress has required a close liaison among the disciplines of chemistry, pharmacology and the clinic—all seeking the elusive relationship between chemical structure and biological action that ordinarily is established only by a carefully contrived laboratory investigation. The handful of active agents culled from the examination of thousands of compounds in many laboratories attests to the complexity of the task.

By analogy with the surgical procedure of sympathectomy, the action of the more specific antihypertensive drugs—typified by guanethidine—has been denoted as a pharmacological sympathectomy. In fact, guanethidine, by virtue of its potency, persistence and specificity, can produce a more encompassing sympathectomy than ever could be achieved surgically, since it involves all the nervous pathways, including those beyond the reach of the surgeon. Moreover, the drug-induced sympathectomy is not irreversible but rather affords the physician the opportunity of adapting the degree and duration of the effect to the needs of the patient.

With the advantage of two decades of research and of steadily improving pharmacological and biochemical methods for assessing potentially useful antihypertensive action, the hope for even more efficient remedies seems promising. This much is known: The reward has been worth the effort, for the cumulative experience issuing from the clinic has been encouraging. With blood pressure lowered, the enlarged heart has returned to normal size; kidney deterioration has been arrested; narrowed vessels of the retina have widened. Thus good health has been restored, and life expectancies lengthened for untold thousands of middle aged and elderly people.

Suggested Reading

Best, C. H., & Taylor, N. B. *The Physiological Basis of Medical Practice.* (8th ed.) Baltimore: Williams and Wilkins, 1966.

Bock, K. D., & Cottier, P. T. Essential Hypertension, an International Symposium, Berne, June 7-10, 1960. Berlin: Springer-Verlag. 1960.

Brest, A. N., & Moyer, J. H. *Hypertension—Recent Advances, The Second Hahnemann Symposium on Hypertensive Disease.* Philadelphia: Lea and Febiger, 1961.

DiPalma, J. R. *Drill's Pharmacology in Medicine.* (3rd ed.) New York: McGraw-Hill, 1965.

deStevens, G. Diuretics—Chemistry and Pharmacology. *Medicinal Chemistry, a Series of Monographs,* New York: Academic Press 1963, *1.*

Genest, J., & Koiw, E. *Hypertension '72*. New York: Springer-Verlag, 1972.

Goodman, L. S., & Gilman, A. *The Pharmacological Basis of Therapeutics*. (3rd ed.) New York: MacMillan, 1965.

Gross, F. *Antihypertensive Therapy—Principles and Practice, an International Symposium*. Berlin: Springer-Verlag, 1966.

Laragh, J. H., Symposium on Hypertension: Mechanisms and Management. *The American Journal of Medicine*, 1972, *52*(5), 565–720.

Mulrow, P. J., Supplement No. II, *Hypertension;* Vol. 28, No. 5, May, 1971 and *Salt, Hormones and Hypertension.* Vol. 19, Circulation Research.

Pickering, W. G. *High Blood Pressure*. London: Churchill, 1955.

Reader, R., (Oxon), F.R.A.C.P., M.R.C.P., Supplement No. II, *Hypertensive Mechanisms*, Vol. 27, No. 4. Circulation Research, October, 1970.

Schlittler, E. Antihypertensive Agents. *Medicinal Chemistry—A Series of Monographs*, New York: Academic Press, 1967, *7*.

Smirk, F. H. *High Arterial Pressure*. Illinois: Springfield, 1957.

Weyer, E. M. New Adrenergic Blocking Agents: Their Pharmacological, Biochemical and Clinical Actions. *Annals of the New York Academy of Sciences*, 1967, *139*, 541–1009.

CHAPTER 8

Biochemical Approaches to Medicinal Research and Development

Mitchell N. Cayen

The living organism is a teeming world of molecules arranged in such a manner that the organism functions in harmony. Disease signals that one or more molecular components is malfunctioning. Hence, an understanding of the organism's functions can lead to a better understanding of the origins of disease. The development of medicines entails the study of the interaction between drug molecules and those of living systems. Biochemistry focuses on the properties of molecules that comprise biological systems, to find out how they function in health and disease.

Biopolymers

Many kinds of molecules are found only in living systems. Among these are the biopolymers—giant molecules built by linkages of simpler molecules. The major biopolymers can be divided into three groups:

1. *Polysaccharides*, the simplest biopolymers, are polymers of simple carbohydrates (sugars). Their biological function is relatively passive. For example, starch and glycogen serve as nutritional reservoirs, and cellulose has mainly a structural role. (See Figure 1.)

2. *Nucleic acids*, linear polymers of nucleotides, consist of a nitrogenous base, a sugar and phosphoric acid. (See Figure 2.) RNA (ribonucleic acid) and DNA (desoxyribonucleic acid) form the code that directs genetic processes and protein synthesis; thus they form the basis of life itself.

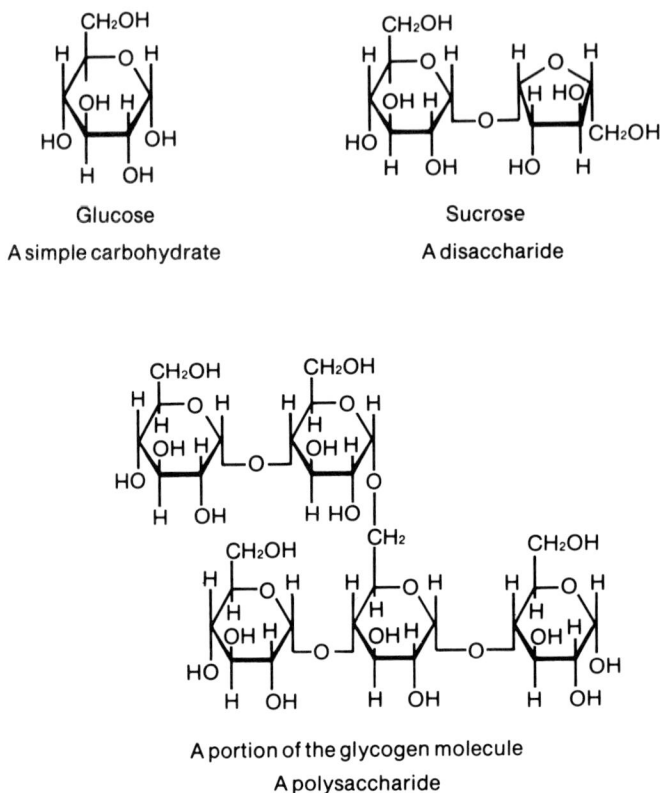

Glucose
A simple carbohydrate

Sucrose
A disaccharide

A portion of the glycogen molecule
A polysaccharide

Figure 1. Carbohydrate structures.

3. *Proteins,* the most prevalent of the biopolymers, play a role in almost all biological activities. They consist of linear polymers of amino acids, which may be cross-linked to form very complex structures. Proteins can be classified into many groups according to their function:

Structural proteins (e.g., collagen and elastin) are relatively inert to biochemical processes. They help to maintain the form and function of various components of living systems, from the largest organs to cellular and subcellular membranes.

Contractile proteins, such as muscle proteins (e.g., myosin and actin) supply the capacity of motion or of external work (e.g., circulation and digestion).

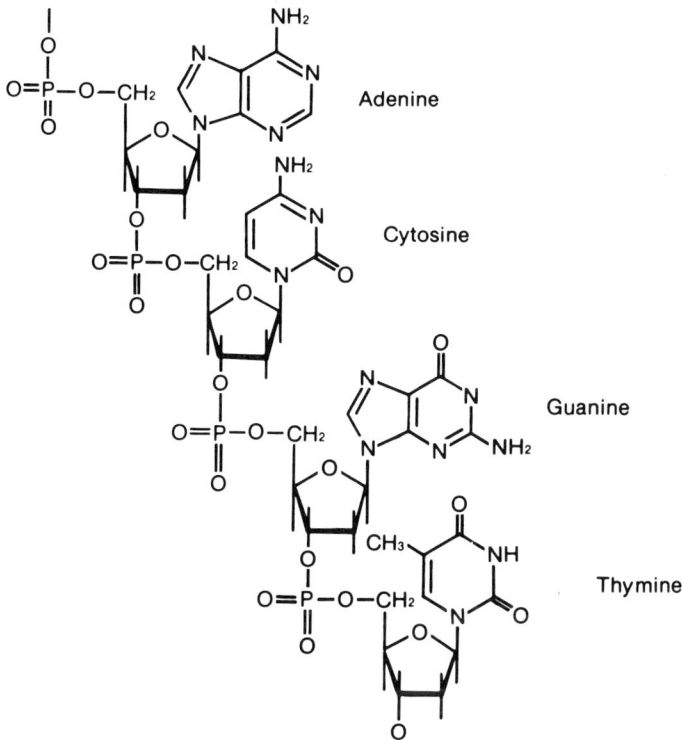

Figure 2. Structure of the polynucleotide chain in DNA.

Transport, or *carrier proteins,* are essential for the transport of biological factors within the organism. For example, hemoglobin transports oxygen, and albumin carries thyroxine, fatty acids and many foreign compounds, such as drugs.

Catalytic proteins, called enzymes, catalyze an extraordinary variety of chemical processes that are vital for normal functioning of living cells.

Enzymes are biological catalysts, effective in small amounts and specific and selective in their action. The materials on which enzymes act are called substrates. A group of enzymes having a particular type of substrate is designated by combining the root of the substrate with the suffix -*ase*; thus an enzyme that acts on a protein is a proteinase, or on ribonucleic acid, a ribonuclease. Enzymes also may be classified according to the reaction catalyzed, so that an enzyme that catalyzes oxidation is an oxidase, and so on. Most enzyme-catalyzed reactions proceed with a delicacy and precision that cannot be matched by classical methods of organic chemistry.

Other groups of proteins include the peptide hormones, such as ACTH, growth hormone and insulin and antibodies, formed by the organism to specifically counteract foreign agents.

Enzymes and Biochemical Screening

The expression *intermediary metabolism* describes the study of the formation and breakdown (biosynthesis and catabolism) of components of living systems. Research in intermediary metabolism has accounted for some of the greatest biochemical achievements over the past 50 years. Results of this research can be summarized in metabolic maps. The metabolic pathways for sugars, fatty acids, amino acids, cholesterol, hormones, nucleic acids and even proteins largely have been mapped.

Many diseases result from a metabolic disorder in which a normal component of an organism is produced at an abnormal rate. A unique aspect of biological systems is that most metabolic conversions are controlled by enzymes. Recognizing this feature, pharmaceutical scientists have used enzymes as targets for controlling disease.

A disease caused by a change in the normal rate of a biochemical transformation may be due to an abnormality of the enzyme that controls the transformation. An ideal drug would be one that controls, without side effects, the enzymatic process involved in the pathogenesis of the disease. Medicines that control enzyme systems combat such conditions as depression, abnormal blood clotting, gout, epilepsy and high blood pressure. (See Chapters 5 and 7.)

The first step in developing a drug that affects biochemical processes is to gain an understanding of the processes and how they respond to various physiological stimuli. For example, in many instances a disease develops when the body produces too much or too little of a normal constituent. Too little insulin triggers diabetes. Too much or too little adrenaline disturbs functioning of the brain and nervous system. Too much stom-

ach acid can cause ulcers, and so on. Administration of the
proper constituents can overcome such deficiencies; this relieves
the symptoms but does not cure the disease.

One approach to the problem: Control the rate of formation
of the body constituent by suppressing or potentiating the
effect of an enzyme involved in its formation. But how? In
what tissue or tissues is the constituent synthesized? What are
the precursors and intermediates in its formation? What enzymes are involved? How does the rate of formation respond to
certain biological stimuli? How much is normally produced? If
produced at an abnormal rate, is this the cause or result of the
disease in question? To achieve the desired result, what would
be the best enzyme to inhibit or stimulate? Dr. George Hitchings of Burroughs Wellcome Co. answered such questions in
research on the control of gout. In this disease hard materials
are deposited on the tissues, especially in the joints. These
materials are mainly insoluble salts of uric acid, which is the end
product of amino acid catabolism. The body eliminates nitrogen
by excreting uric acid in urine. When too much uric acid
accumulates or when its elimination is abnormal due to a
kidney problem, the soluble uric acid forms insoluble solid salts
(urates); these collect in various tissues and cause the painful
symptoms of gout.

Dr. Hitchings approached the problem by focusing on the
intermediary metabolism of uric acid. The immediate precursor
of uric acid is the purine called xanthine. The conversion of
xanthine to uric acid is catalyzed by the enzyme xanthine
oxidase. Dr. Hitchings and his associates searched for a drug
that would inhibit xanthine oxidase, thereby reducing the formation of uric acid. Their search was successful, and today
allopurinol effectively controls gout.

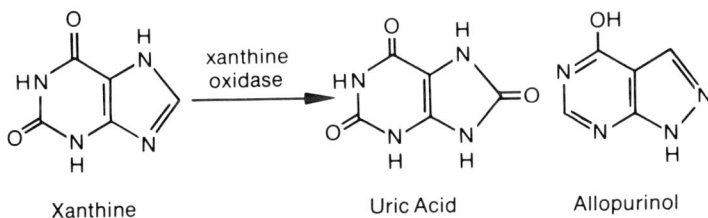

Xanthine   Uric Acid   Allopurinol

In a research program based on a biochemical rationale, the medicinal chemist synthesizes compounds that he believes will have the best chance of affecting the biochemical process in question. Each compound undergoes one or more screenings— routine assays designed to give specific data on how it affects the process in question. When feasible, an isolated tissue or enzyme from an experimental animal is treated with the compound *in vitro* and the effect measured on the formation of the desired end-product. Thus scientists discovered the activity of allopurinol as a result of a screen for xanthine oxidase inhibition. *In vitro* assays permit researchers to test many compounds in a short time and to obtain data quickly on a specific reaction in a given tissue. Since most metabolic reactions take place in the liver, this organ frequently is removed from the animal and tested in a suitable medium with the appropriate substrate. Other tissues used for *in vitro* screening tests include brain homogenates, fat tissue, stomach, intestine, lung, etc.

In the search for a drug that will have a biological effect resulting from direct action on a given enzyme, compounds are first tested *in vitro* in the isolated tissue enzyme system. Active compounds are then submitted to *in vivo* testing to measure their effect on the given enzyme in the intact animal. Although many factors come into play when a compound is administered to whole animals, the correlation between *in vitro* and *in vivo* data is often direct. Compounds that are active *in vivo* may become candidate drugs, if they can satisfy the criteria for safety. On the other hand, agents active *in vitro* may fail *in vivo*. They may never reach the site of action in sufficient amounts. They may decompose to inactive catabolites. They may be too toxic. Such compounds, of course, disappear as potential medicines.

Compounds that are inactive *in vitro* sometimes produce the desired biological action *in vivo* by some means other than that of affecting the enzyme in question. This also complicates research for the biochemist, since the action may be indirect and may be apparent only in the whole animal. For example, clofibrate lowers blood cholesterol levels and suppresses cholesterol biosynthesis in the liver but does not alter the biosynthesis of cholesterol when it is added to a liver homogenate preparation. That is, it is active *in vivo* but not *in vitro*. In spite of deficiencies, *in vitro* screens continue to be widely used for rapid testing of potential drugs.

Drug Activity

Medicines can be designed either to cure a given disease or to alleviate its symptoms. Therapy mitigates many ailments, but cures have been achieved only with antibacterial agents for infectious diseases. Most other drugs elicit only specific responses that moderate symptoms.

Biochemical principles are used not only in the search for new agents but also in evaluating their biological fate in the body—a major element that contributes to drug response. Such studies form the basis for determining optimum dosage, mode and frequency of administration and other factors related to drug therapy. Three phases of drug activity can be differentiated: (a) the pharmaceutical phase, in which the drug is administered and released in a dispersed form from a pharmaceutical preparation; (b) the pharmacokinetic phase, which involves absorption, distribution, metabolism and excretion; and (c) the pharmacodynamic phase, which is concerned with the uptake of the drug at the target organ and the actual therapeutic response. (See Figure 3.)

Phases of Drug Activity

Pharmaceutical Phase

To be effective, a medicine must reach its site of action. Unless it acts topically (at the site of application), it must first be transported by the blood stream to its site of action.

Preferred routes of drug administration may be divided into two classes—oral and parenteral. In the oral route, the drug reaches the gastrointestinal (GI) tract by mouth (tablet, capsule or as part of the diet or drinking water). The parenteral method bypasses the GI tract, and is effected by subcutaneous, intra-

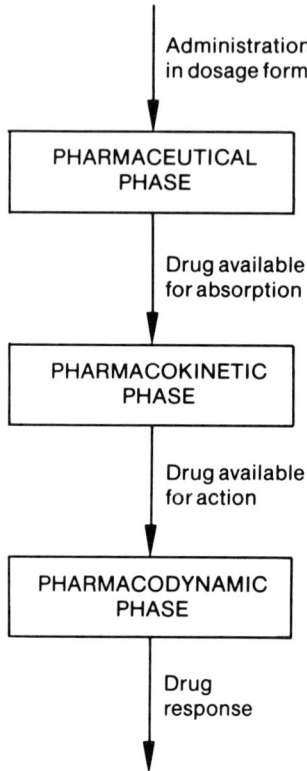

Figure 3. Phases of drug activity.

muscular or intravenous injection, by topical application to the
skin, by inhalation or by other routes, such as intravaginal or
rectal administration.

The desired mode of action and chemistry of the drug sometimes dictate the mode of administration. Doctors and patients
usually prefer the oral route. However, if a drug is not absorbed
or if it is altered in the GI tract (e.g., insulin, morphine and
certain penicillins), it will fail to reach its site of action. An
empty stomach caters to gastric absorption in which the drug,
unimpeded by food, will have easy access to the mucosal wall.
A doctor often recommends that his patient take a medicine

with or after a meal if it irritates the gastric mucosa. In other instances, food may facilitate absorption. For example, fat in the diet aids absorption of the antifungal agent griseofulvin.

The biochemist studies factors that govern absorption of drugs from the GI tract, which are based on chemical and physical properties. From these evaluations he tries to predict the chances of a compound to voyage successfully through the GI wall. Drugs intended for action within the GI tract, however, are not designed to be absorbed and must be given orally—for instance, an antimicrobial drug designed to act on certain unwanted bacteria in the intestine. For this drug to be absorbed and thereby removed from its site of action would be undesirable. On the other hand, minor chemical modifications of the sulfonamide antibiotics have changed them from nonabsorbable to absorbable antibacterial drugs useful for treating infections elsewhere in the body.

The way a drug is prepared, i.e., its formulation, can drastically affect its biological activity after oral administration. If manufactured in such a way that it is not absorbed, then it will have no biological activity (assuming, of course, that it does not act in the GI tract). The science of *biopharmaceutics* deals with the relationships between the chemical and physical properties of a drug and components with which it is combined to formulate a dosage form.

Physical properties, of course, can affect absorption. A drug may exist as two or more crystal forms that are chemically identical but dissolve at different rates in the GI tract. The one that goes into solution most rapidly is more likely to produce swift and consistent responses. For example, crystalline forms of the antibiotics novobiocin and chloramphenicol are inert, while the GI tract readily absorbs the amorphous forms, which then produce the required response. Particle size also plays a role, as with the antifungal drug griseofulvin; the smaller the particles, the more drug is absorbed, because of greater surface areas. If aspirin is properly mixed with antacids and granulated with starch, absorption improves. Different drug preparations containing the same active principle help the patient in some instances and have little or no effect in others. Differences in formulation often mean differences in response.

A drug injected intravenously into the blood stream provides the advantages of minimum delay (in acute or emergency situations) and maximum control. Large amounts of fluid can be introduced over a long time by a constant infusion apparatus, thus accurately controlling a drug's blood level. Intravenous injection suits substances that do not lend themselves to oral entry. Also, medicines that would be painful in subcutaneous or muscle tissues often may be slowly injected intravenously—for example, nitrogen mustard used in cancer chemotherapy.

The intramuscular or subcutaneous route is used when a drug is not absorbed intact from the GI tract and when there is no need for direct entry into the blood. Small molecules are absorbed directly into the capillaries from an intramuscular site, while larger molecules, such as protein, gain access to the circulation by means of the lymphatic channels.

Drug Metabolism and the Pharmacokinetic Phase

The past 30 years have witnessed the golden age of medicinal introductions, during which more than 1,000 new single-entity drugs have been marketed in North America. Today, increasing difficulties confront new drug development, not only because of enhanced demands for efficacy and safety but because of a decline in the number of basic approaches aimed at the amelioration of disease. Many present-day afflictions of our advanced society (e.g., cardiovascular disease, diabetes, malignant tumors, mental illness, inflammatory diseases—such as arthritis and rheumatism) require prolonged therapy lasting for months or years—in marked contrast to the short, intensive therapy required for the treatment of infectious diseases. For these reasons drug development has become more sophisticated, a fact exemplified by the field of drug metabolism.

The purpose of drug metabolism studies is to determine the metabolic fate of a medicine after it enters the body; the goal is to find out how the patient can attain optimum benefit and safety. Metabolic studies have become integral to preclinical and clinical evaluation of new drugs.

Such studies measure rates and sites of absorption, blood and tissue levels of the drug and its metabolites, half-life (a measure of the rate of disappearance of drug from the blood), protein-binding, rate of metabolism, rate and route of excretion, entero-hepatic circulation (i.e., circulation through the liver), tissue accumulation, placental transfer, interaction with other drugs, isolation and identification of metabolites. Many of these parameters can be defined in mathematical terms, and the science of pharmacokinetics uses mathematical methods to define the metabolic disposition of a drug.

Two approaches, of fundamental importance in drug metabolism, are based on (a) the availability of sophisticated and sensitive instrumentation to distinguish between low levels of the drug and its metabolites, and (b) the use of radioactive tracers.

Since a metabolite generally differs from its precursor by only a single chemical change, the need for sophisticated and sensitive *instrumentation* that can separate metabolites—and which can distinguish between the unchanged drug and its metabolites—is imperative in drug metabolism studies and for the development of valid pharmacokinetic data. Instruments such as the autoanalyzer, spectrophotometer, fluorimeter and gas chromatograph enable the analytical measurement and detection of extremely low levels of unchanged drug and its metabolites in blood, urine and various tissues.

Spectroscopy techniques such as infrared, ultraviolet and nuclear magnetic resonance, as well as mass spectrometry, are employed in the qualitative determination of a metabolite's molecular structure once it has been isolated in pure form.

Radioactive tracers have revolutionized many aspects of biochemistry and pharmaceutical research. Their use is based on the principle that all forms of a compound—whether radioactive or not—have identical chemical or biological properties.

Radioactive carbon (C^{14}) and hydrogen (H^3 or tritium) are weak beta emitters; that is, they release electrons of low energy and thus are not harmful to living systems. Since most drugs and molecules of biological origin contain carbon and hydrogen, these substances lend themselves to labeling with C^{14} or H^3.

Less frequently, other radioactive elements such as S^{35}, I^{131} or P^{32} are used for labeling, but these are special cases.

Radioactivity provides a compound with an identification tag or label. The radioisotope can be distinguished from nonradioactive materials simply by measuring the amount of radioactivity present with detectors. Such devices for measuring radioactivity are more sensitive than most other analytical techniques and instruments. Radioactivity sensors can detect as little as one-trillionth of a gram (a "picogram") of a compound—a virtually impossible achievement for compounds that are not radioactive.

Applications of radiotracer technology appear to be limited only by the imagination of the medicinal scientist. Radioactive tracers used in certain *in vitro* screening programs attain an accuracy and efficiency that would be impossible without them.

The measurement of cholesterol biosynthesis *in vitro* by rat liver preparations exemplies this technique. High blood cholesterol levels long have been correlated with many heart and circulatory diseases, such as atherosclerosis. The origin of blood cholesterol is twofold: diet and biosynthesis in such tissues as the liver and intestinal wall. Development of a drug that would inhibit cholesterol biosynthesis without side effects had at one time been conceived as an approach to the lowering of blood cholesterol levels. To develop this idea, it was first necessary to elucidate the intermediary metabolism of cholesterol. This has been worked out, and it is now known that the main precursor of cholesterol is acetate. In the *in vitro* screening program, radioactive acetate (acetate-C^{14}) is incubated with a rat liver preparation in the presence of the test compound; then the amount of radioactive cholesterol (cholesterol-C^{14}) formed is measured. If less cholesterol-C^{14} is produced in the presence of, rather than in the absence of the test substance, the compound could become a candidate for study as a potential cholesterol-lowering agent.

Radiotracer techniques often provide the only practical means of detecting the small amounts of compounds involved in drug metabolism studies. A radioactive drug's absorption, distribution, metabolism and elimination can be determined by measuring its radioactivity and its metabolites in blood, tissues, urine and feces. The difference between the concentration of unchanged drugs (as determined by a specific analytical technique) and compounds derived from total radioactivity in a sample is due to metabolite(s) of the drug.

More than any other new technique, isotopic labeling has helped to transform the study of drug metabolism from a semiquantitative to a fully quantitative discipline. Such an advance has opened new fields of study, including those concerned with agents that affect the brain.

The central nervous system is unique among biological tissues for many reasons, among them the property known as the blood-brain barrier. Its peculiar membranes separate the cells of nervous tissue from innervating capillaries. Unlike those of other organs, these membranes are permeable only to specific types of molecules and so protect sensitive nervous tissue cells from harmful agents. This property poses a problem in drug research, because many candidate drugs designed to act on the brain will not pass the blood-brain barrier. Studies of how a drug penetrates the blood-brain barrier and how it is localized in certain cells are facilitated by tissue section autoradiography, a radiotracer technique that traces the fate of a labeled drug by exposing brain sections to X-ray film.

Autoradiography also measures *tissue distribution* of radioactivity throughout the animal. The technique, called whole body autoradiography qualitatively determines the rate of uptake and disappearance of radioactivity in different organs of the body. Rodents (rats or mice) are given the radioactive drug and are killed by rapid freezing at various times after dosing. They are then imbedded into blocks of ice containing carboxymethylcellulose. Housed in a refrigerated chamber, the block is mounted on a microtome, which hydraulically cuts cross-sectionally thin slices (20 microns) through various levels of the carcass. (See Figure 4.) The slice is then exposed to X-ray film for 4 to 6 weeks, and the various intensities of grey areas on the resultant autoradiogram give a pictorial qualitative estimate of the amount of radioactivity in various organs. (See Figure 5.)

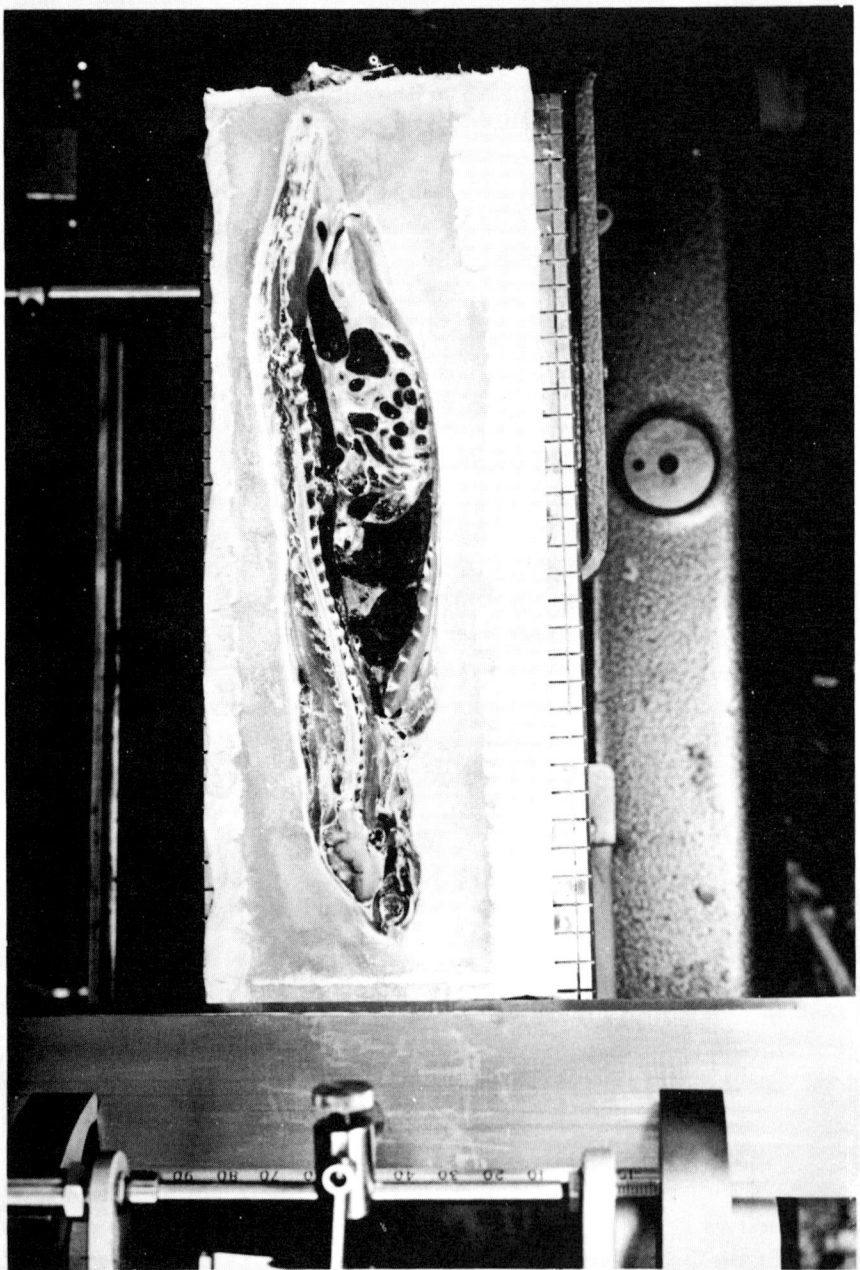

Figure 24 Autoradiography. This slice of frozen carcass of a rat being cut in a refrigerated chamber

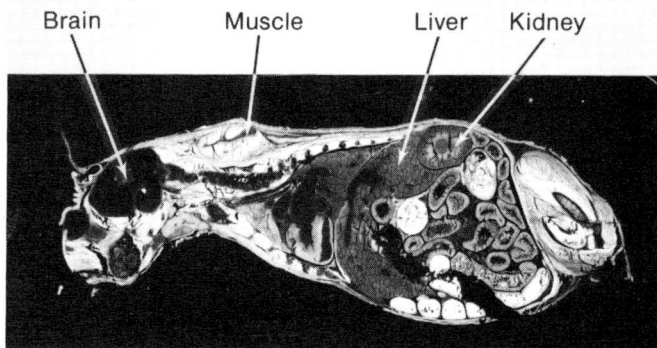

Figure 5. Autoradiogram shows the distribution of an experimental drug (light areas) in the different organs of a mouse. Note the presence of drug in muscle, kidney and liver and absence of drug in brain.

To obtain a quantitative measurement of radioactivity in certain tissues, a portion of the tissue can be solubilized in strong alkali or can be burned so that radioactivity is emitted as $[^{14}C]O_2$ or $[^3H]_2O$, which is subsequently trapped. In both methods, liquid scintillation spectrophotometry measures the radioactivity content.

Once they reach the blood, most medicines are distributed throughout the body in the water phase of blood plasma. The uptake of a drug by a tissue or organ depends on the rate of blood flow and the rate at which drug molecules enter into the cells of that organ. Some drugs may be bound to plasma proteins and thus do not freely diffuse out of the plasma.

The amount of a medicine present in a given tissue is usually a very small proportion of the total in the body. The site of action may be associated with a subcellular component within the target organ. Often, a minor chemical modification increases drug bioavailability, that is, increases uptake by the target organ. Thus, tissue distribution studies can aid in the development of superior medications.

Metabolism, accumulation in tissues and excretion eliminate the drug from the circulation. The rate of each of these processes that terminate drug action is determined by chemical and physical properties of the drug, its combination with target organs and its interaction with the tissues responsible for its elimination. The kidney plays a key role in drug excretion. Some medicines are excreted into the GI tract directly from the blood or by way of the bile. Others may be partially eliminated through the lungs or the skin. Usually, compounds with a low molecular weight are excreted mainly in the urine, while the biliary route becomes important with higher molecular weights. Certain agents may accumulate in specific tissues. For example, fat-soluble drugs may settle in the large depots of body fat where they exert no biological activity.

Most medicines are lipid soluble rather than water soluble and therefore must be converted into water soluble metabolites in order to be excreted. It may be asked why drugs should be metabolized at all; why can't they be excreted in the kidneys (or with bile into the feces) like other unwanted compounds? Evolution provides an answer. Fish do not possess enzymes capable of metabolizing drugs or foreign compounds; they are not needed because water washes the gills continuously and therefore readily removes foreign compounds, even those that diffuse poorly.

The adaptation to terrestrial life depended on efficient mechanisms for the conservation of water and the development of a highly organized kidney. This created a new problem, because the kidney could not excrete highly lipid soluble compounds. These substances become strongly bound to tissues; in fact, pharmacokinetic equations calculate that if certain lipid soluble drugs were not metabolized, their half-life (i.e., time required for body levels of a compound to decrease to one-half of a previous level) would be in the order of 100 years. Overdosage, therefore, could bring about permanent intoxication. Dr. Bernard Brodie of the National Institutes of Health has likened the fate of a nonmetabolized lipid soluble drug to the Flying Dutchman, doomed to roam the seas of life forever. Metabolism of these drugs to water soluble metabolites can be viewed as a means of terminating drug action. Water soluble drugs do not need to be metabolized and are very often excreted unchanged.

Drugs are metabolized mainly in the liver and to a lesser extent in such tissues as lungs, kidneys and walls of the GI tract. Drug transformations can be divided into two categories. In phase 1, reactions (biotransformations) include hydroxylations, oxidations, reductions and hydrolysis, i.e., enzymatic reactions in which a new functional group is introduced into the drug molecule or an existing functional group is modified. In phase 2, reactions are conjugations, which are enzymatic syntheses whereby a functional group is masked by addition of a new group, such as glucuronic acid, sulfate, methyl, acetyl or certain amino acids. The ultimate purpose of these metabolic transformations is to bring about elimination of the drug. The isolation and identification of metabolites comprise an integral part of defining a drug's biological fate.

Aside from having the required pharmacological activity, the ideal drug should have the following characteristics: It should (a) reach the site of action, (b) arrive at the site rapidly and in sufficient quantity, (c) remain for a sufficient duration of time, (d) be excluded from other sites, and (e) eventually be removed from the site and from the body. Pharmacokinetics is concerned with quantitatively accounting for the whereabouts of a drug after it has been introduced into the body, with analysis carried out throughout the entire time course. By analyzing accessible biological materials (blood, urine, feces), mathematical derivations delineate the amount of drug and metabolites in non-accessible regions, perhaps even the site of action. Such kinetic data aid in evaluating how close the medicine approaches the ideal and can provide valuable information toward the design of superior agents.

Figure 6 depicts some of the factors of pharmacokinetic analyses. Most drugs must first enter the blood before reaching the site of action. Certain ones are highly bound to blood protein; they may prolong drug action, since in most instances only the unbound drug creates biological activity. The equilibrium characteristics of the drug in blood at the receptor site, in the storage depot and in other tissues can be expressed by various rate constants. Rate constants also define absorption, blood level, volume of distribution, protein-binding, rate of

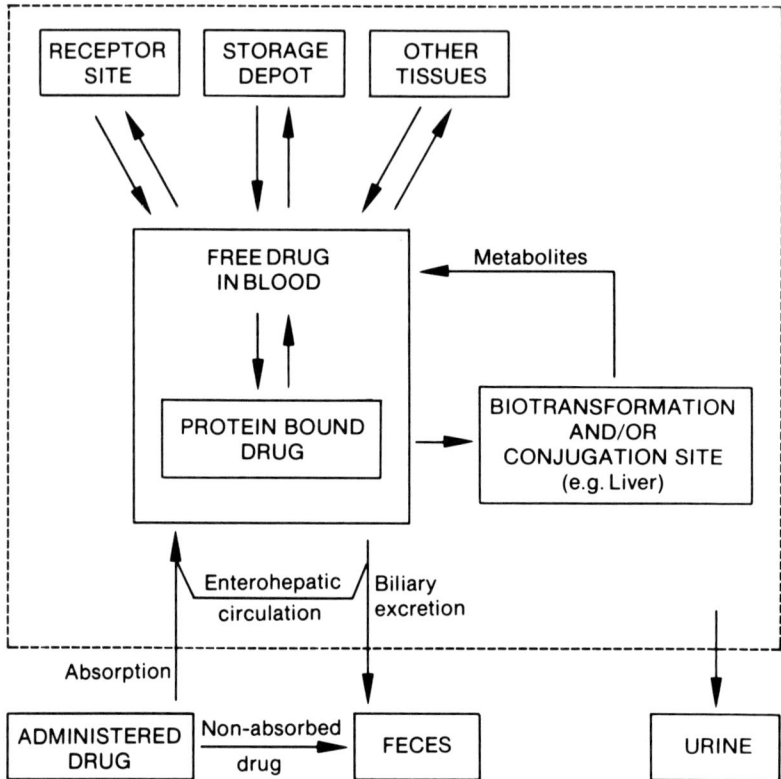

Figure 6. Pharmacokinetics: factors which regulate body levels and time-course of pharmacological effects of drugs.

biotransformation and conjugation, renal clearance and urinary excretion, fecal excretion, biliary excretion, enterohepatic circulation (i.e., drug and/or metabolites excreted via the bile into the GI tract and subsequently reabsorbed), etc.

The metabolic disposition of a drug is not only a characteristic of the drug itself but also is affected by various physiological and environmental factors. The very young and very old have altered metabolism. The rate of metabolism also may vary by sex. Nutrition, stress, trauma, pregnancy, fever and certain disease can markedly affect metabolic profiles. The size and

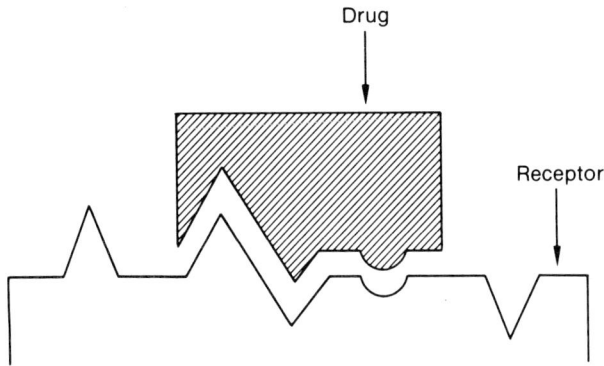

Figure 7. Schematic diagram of receptor site and substrate (drug).

frequency of dose will often affect metabolism and pharma-cokinetics. (The effects of drug interactions and genetic factors will be covered later in this chapter.)

Pharmacodynamics: Drug Design and Receptors

Now that we have discussed testing of drugs and the first two phases of drug activity from the biochemical point of view, let us go back to the beginning to probe the broader implications of drug design. What has the biochemist learned about control of biological activity at the molecular level that can be applied to develop a superior medicine?

He has learned that the biological action of a drug (or, for that matter, of a normal body constituent) results from physio-chemical interaction with functionally important molecules in the organism. The site where all this action takes place is called a receptor.

In most cases the receptor is a site on a biopolymer. Orig-inally, scientists believed that a drug could combine with one and only one receptor in a lock-and-key fashion. (See Figure 7.) This concept of the drug-receptor combination, although still generally accepted, has been refined in recent years. A drug-receptor interaction can involve bonding interactions of various types, such as covalent bonds, hydrogen bonds, ionic bonds and hydrophobic interactions.

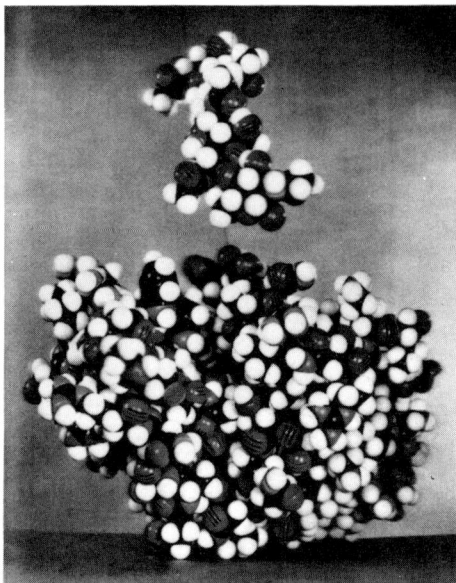

Figure 8. Enzyme model. Substrate poised above the active site of lysozyme.

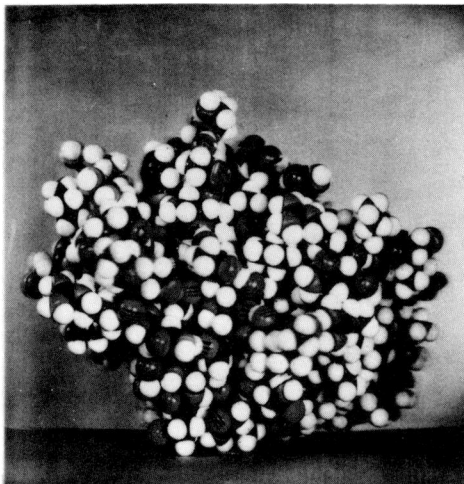

Figure 9. Enzyme-substrate interaction. The substrate of Figure 8 fills the active site of the enzyme.

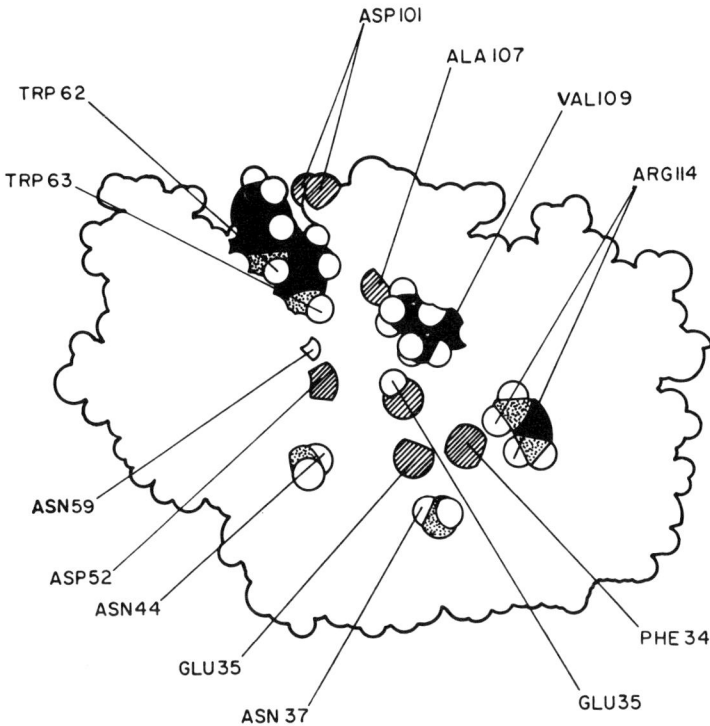

Figure 10. Elements of the active site. Carbon atoms are black and hydrogens are white in this sketch and in Figure 8. Nitrogens that are light gray in Figure 8 are stippled in the sketch and oxygens that are dark gray in Figure 8 are diagonally shaded. The hydrogens that are participate in hydrogen bonds with substrate are specified by the points of termination of identifying lines. Figures 8, 9 and 10 have been adapted from R. A. Harte and J. N. Rupley, "Three-dimensional Pictures of Molecular Models" in *The Journal of Biological Chemistry*, Vol. 243, pp. 1663-1669 (1968). The original article contains magnificant three-dimensional pictures in full color.

Most drugs interact with a receptor by means of a combination of numerous bonds of several types, causing the lock-and-key effect. The interactions produce a change in biological activity and are reversible so that the drug does not act for an exceedingly long time.

An important step in developing the ideal medicine is to provide a concept about receptors. We have seen the fruits of such concepts in Chapter 7. It would be most useful, of course, if we could identify, isolate and characterize the receptor with which the drug will interact.

Scientists are making great progress toward the isolation and characterization of pharmacological receptor sites. In the meantime, they have learned much by studying the interactions of enzymes and their substrates.

For example, Dr. C. C. F. Blake and Dr. D. C. Phillips and their associates at the Royal Institution in London have used X-ray crystallography to study the interaction of the hexamer of N-acetyl glucosamine with the enzyme lysozyme. This enzyme functions in higher organisms to provide a powerful defensive mechanism against a large group of bacteria. The natural substrate of lysozyme in the living organism is a sugar polymer in the bacterial cell wall which is cleaved by the enzyme. The hexamer of N-acetylglucosamine resembles a portion of the natural substrate. Dr. Phillips and his co-workers have shown that the hexamer fits neatly into a cleft which is the active site of the enzyme. The resulting enzyme-substrate complex has many hydrogen bonds.

Figure 8 is a photograph of a space filling model of the substrate poised above the active site cavity of a model of the lysozyme molecule. In Figure 9 the substrate fills the cavity and forms hydrogen bonds with the enzyme. Some of these hydrogen bonds may be located with the help of Figure 10. The original photographs corresponding to Figures 8 and 9 are "Xographs" which appear in color and in three dimensions. They show with remarkable clarity just how fine the fit can be between an enzyme and its substrate. From studies of the structure-activity relationships of compounds closely related to drugs we know that many of them have features that must be very narrowly defined to fit the pharmacological receptor and provide the desired activity.

Since enzymes, as catalysts, regulate the rate of metabolic reactions, much concerted effort has focused on these proteins in studying drug-receptor reactions and the properties of the receptor itself. Ribonuclease is a classic example. This enzyme catalyzes the catabolism of RNA and thus is vital to life processes. The structure and spatial design of pancreatic ribonuclease has been completely elucidated; it is the first and, to date, the only enzyme that has been chemically synthesized from its component amino acids. As for the nucleic acids themselves, combined efforts of chemists, biochemists and geneticists have clarified the structure and spatial design of these biopolymers and hence made clear how nucleic acids direct protein synthesis. Sophisticated separation techniques are being used to isolate receptors in pure form from target organs.

Such success stories open the door for understanding drug actions. We stand on the threshhold of an era in which we will comprehend how the interaction of bonds between polymer receptor (the lock) and drug (the key) modifies the biopolymer function in such a way as to produce characteristic drug action.

Usually, medicinal research has had to rely on inferences drawn about a receptor by systematically testing a series of compounds. A series of structure-activity relationships is formulated. A biological effect is chosen, and from the information available about structure-activity relations, researchers synthesize and test a prototype compound. They modify its molecular structure by adding, removing or altering one or more substituents. These chemically related compounds, in turn, are tested. After the researchers compare the biological potency of each member of the series, conclusions emerge about the precise mode by which a drug combines with a receptor site. They may find, for example, that the receptor binds only a certain part of the molecule and that minor modifications of the remaining portions of the molecule may reduce toxicity, increase absorption from the GI tract, prolong drug action, increase potency or alter passage through the blood-brain barrier. This trial-and-error approach has proved to be valuable in the past and should continue to play a major role in the future. However, we are seeing fewer errors and more trials as our insight into drug-receptor interaction increases.

There are many ways in which the study of drug-receptor interactions has increased our understanding of how drugs act.

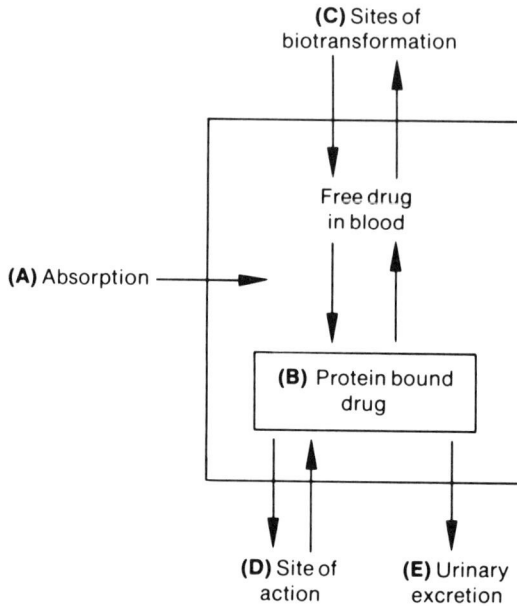

Figure 11. Some sites at which drugs may interact in the body.

Some drugs alter membrane function to permit a change in permeability to ions. Some are competitive inhibitors, i.e., drugs compete with a normal body constituent for the same receptor site, for example, on an enzyme, thus preventing or hindering the biological action of this constituent. A drug may cause enzyme induction; this is based on the principle that the enzyme content of a tissue is maintained by equal rates of enzyme synthesis and degradation and that an agent that increases the former or decreases the latter causes a rise in tissue enzyme level. This results in a stepped-up rate of the metabolic reaction that is catalyzed by this enzyme.

Drug Interaction

Multiple drug therapy, as we know, is commonplace in modern medicine. In the course of a patient's illness, his doctor may prescribe many medicines simultaneously. Not uncommonly, many unusual symptoms may appear. Because of a lack of an adequate explanation, they could be ignored or attributed to an unusual manifestation of the disease itself. Only within recent years has it become evident that one drug may affect the action of another.

Such reactions may diminish or abolish the intended beneficial effects of one or both medicines or they may enhance the activity of one or both, or produce an undesirable side effect or toxic manifestation not associated with the respective products individually.

Drugs as chemicals can react with each other outside the organism. However, when two or more drugs are ingested, many possibilities for interactions occur. Figure 11 depicts some of them.

Absorption

Within the GI tract, a large number of possible interactions reduce drug absorption. For example, tetracycline antibiotics form poorly absorbed chelates with calcium, iron and magnesium ions; concurrent use of antacids containing these ions (or milk, which contains calcium) will reduce the absorption of tetracycline. Cholestyramine, a nonabsorbable ion exchange resin, binds bile acids in the GI tract; as bile acids are required for the absorption of cholesterol, the resin becomes a cholesterol-lowering agent. Since cholestyramine also binds acidic drugs such as aspirin, concurrent administration of cholestyramine and certain acidic agents will inhibit absorption.

Protein Binding

Many medicines are insoluble in blood. They circulate throughout the blood bound to plasma proteins, mainly to albumin. A drug bound to plasma albumin does not diffuse to the active receptor site, but stays, however, in equilibrium with the free (i.e., active) form. If drugs A and B are strongly bound to albumin, their administration will result in a competition for the albumin binding sites, or drug A may displace drug B from albumin and produce toxic side effects due to apparent overdosage of drug B. When warfarin (an anticoagulant) and phenylbutazone (an anti-inflammatory) are given together, these highly bound agents induce a release of warfarin from plasma albumin and cause bleeding. Aspirin can displace protein-bound penicillin analogues or long acting sulfonamides.

Biotransformation

Certain drugs can stimulate the biotransformation of others; on repeated dosing they can also inhibit their own biotransformation. The process, called enzyme induction, results from the drug-induced increase in liver microsomal enzyme activity. Since drug biotransformation takes place mainly in liver microsomes, enhanced enzyme activity causes an increased rate of drug metabolism. Phenobarbital, griseofulvin and meprobamate are typical enzyme inducers. Great care must be exercised in adjusting doses of enzyme inducers and concommitantly administered medicines. Hence if a patient receives optimum doses of both phenobarbital and warfarin and then spontaneously stops taking phenobarbital, his effective available dose of warfarin will increase (since the rate of degradation is no longer as rapid as in the presence of the inducer), and bleeding may occur.

Site of Action

Drugs can interact at the receptor site to alter the pharmacological response of one or all of them. Such action at receptor sites may be explained in the same manner as substrate-enzyme activity. Thus competitive inhibition may occur when two medicines compete for the same receptor site. Interactions also can occur when an agent or drug acts on another site, either producing an opposite effect or blocking the effect of the drug.

Urinary Excretion

Urinary excretion of compounds involves three processes: passive glomerular filtration, active tubular excretion and passive tubular reabsorption. Active tubular secretion is the transport of the drug from the blood into tubular urine against a concentration gradient. Medicines excreted in this manner include the penicillins, aspirin, phenylbutazone, thiazide diuretics and indomethacin. Excretion rates are altered when drugs compete for the active tubular transport system. Excretion can also be affected by altering the pH of the urine. The diuretic acetazolamide, because of its ability to alkalinize the urine, enhances the excretion of acidic drugs such as aspirin.

Toxicity

Poisonous or toxic properties of medicines must always be examined in detail. Virtually all possess at least some toxicity. Philippus Paracelsus (1493-1541), a professor at the University of Basel, wrote: "All things are poisons, for there is nothing without poisonous qualities. It is only the dose which makes a thing a poison." All drugs are toxic, of course, in overdosage. A common example is the barbiturates. The medicinal scientist must determine correct dose and frequency of administration to elicit the desired effect without toxicity.

Sometimes a toxic effect is an extension of the desired effect at a higher dose level. For example, coumarin anticoagulants prolong the clotting time of blood. Overdosage can lead to a bleeding tendency from excessive prolongation of the clotting time. On the other hand, toxicity often takes the form of a side effect more or less unrelated to primary drug action. Many drugs cause GI disturbances that initiate nausea, vomiting or diarrhea. These occur before the drug is absorbed and reaches its site of action.

In studying drug toxicity in animals, the medicinal scientist uses certain criteria in relating effectiveness and toxicity. One, median effective dose (ED_{50}), is the minimum dose needed to produce a specific effect in 50 percent of the animals. Another, median lethal dose (LD_{50}), is the minimum dose that will cause death in 50 percent of the animals. The wider the range between the lethal and effective doses, the safer the drug is likely to be. This, of course, does not take into account medicines that cause nonlethal side effects. In such cases, the scientist must weigh the seriousness of the disease, the benefit likely to be derived from a given drug and the extent of discomfort or damage which may result from drug toxicity or side effect.

Thus, evaluation of drug activity provides the researcher clues that can lead to the development of improved products. Slight changes in chemical structure may enhance efficacy and safety. These improvements may take the form of increasing absorption from the GI tract, altering the duration of action, changing the rate of metabolism or excretion or decreasing toxic or side effects. The aim of drug development is to produce the ideal medicine, i.e., one that has a selective biological action with the fewest possible side effects and the least possible toxicity.

Molecular Biology

As knowledge about the origins of disease accumulates, the medicinal scientist has become aware of the necessity for a deeper and more complex understanding of biological systems. This need has given rise to molecular biology, the study of biological events at the molecular level in consonance with established principles of chemistry and physics. Especially since the identification of the genetic material as DNA and RNA, molecule biology has mushroomed into an exploding science and become fundamental to medicinal research.

Major discoveries are being made steadily as to how genes control life processes. Subtle differences in the nitrogenous base and spatial design of DNA and RNA molecules can determine whether an organism develops into a dog or a frog. The relationship between genes—the units of heredity—and enzymes—the units of biochemical catalysis—has created a happy marriage between genetics and biochemistry. Genes direct protein synthesis, so biochemical processes in all organisms come under genetic control. Many diseases in man are inherited because of a particular abnormality of a given gene. These inborn errors of metabolism manifest themselves in various ways. For example, a physiologically essential substance may be missing, as in hemophilia; an essential enzymatic activity may be reduced or absent, as in phenylketonuria; an abnormal protein may be present, as in sickle cell anemia; or an alteration may occur in cellular transport of a metabolite, as in cystinuria.

Man and other vertebrates possess a natural defense mechanism to combat diseases caused by foreign bacteria. When a foreign organism challenges the body, specific proteins combine to attack and destroy the invader. These proteins, called antibodies, muster an immunological response. This mechanism protects the body from unwanted bacteria in the environment. Such protection takes several days to develop but once present usually lasts a long time. Antibody development forms the basis for many vaccines, in which the body is pre-sensitized with an attenuated form of the invader. The antibodies remain to combat a later attack by the live form of the bacteria.

Progress in immunology and the genetic control of disease has opened new horizons for the molecular biologist. These new vistas are creating new concepts for the design of drugs to fight disease at the molecular level. Medicines that affect genetic expression, enzyme control and immunological reactions may revolutionize medicinal science once we have learned more about the role of the gene and the antibody in health and disease.

The science of molecular biology also focuses on individual differences in drug response due to genetic variation. These pharmacogenetic studies have shown that there exists marked individual variation in the rate of drug metabolism, in various pharmacokinetic parameters, in the pattern of drug metabolites and in the response of drugs—all of which depend in part on the patient's unique genetic constitution. It has been suggested that each individual has a characteristic rate of drug metabolism, depending on his genetic makeup and his environment. Minor changes in enzyme structure can markedly alter the rate of drug biotransformation and conjugation. Structural modification of serum albumin could produce different binding affinities and alter the fraction of unbound drug (i.e., drug available for action) in the blood.

Pharmacogenetic influences on drug action have been observed by comparing twins. For example, the metabolic disposition of dicumarol (an anticoagulant), antipyrine (an analgesic) and phenylbutazone (an anti-inflammatory) have been studied in various sets of identical as well as fraternal twins. By measuring the rate at which medicines disappear from the blood, it has been revealed that the half lives have much less variance between pairs of identical twins than between pairs of fraternal twins.

Conclusion

At the turn of the century, Dr. Paul Ehrlich summarized his views as follows, "Antitoxins and antibacterial substances are, so to speak, charmed bullets which strike only those objects for whose destruction they have been produced." This dream of a drug that would act at its intended site without any toxicity or side effect has yet to be realized. Still, the study of biological functions at the chemical, physical and molecular levels can lead the way to the development of superior medicines in an effort to realize Ehrlich's dream. The trail has been blazed, and there is room for scientists with uncommon intelligence, foresight and imagination to help broaden these trails into superhighways. The rewards are immeasurable, since the ultimate goal is nothing less than to prevent and cure the diseases that afflict mankind.

> Man consists of body, mind and imagination.
> His body is faulty, his mind untrustworthy,
> but his imagination has made him remarkable.
>
> John Masefield
> (Shakespeare and Spiritual Life)

Suggested Reading

Abrams, W. B. Introducing a New Drug into Clinical Practice. *Anesthesiology*, 1971, *35*, 176–192.

Brodie, B. B., & Heller, W. M. *Bioavailability of Drugs.* New York: S. Karger, 1972. [Originally published: *Pharmacology*, 1972, *8*, (1–3).]

DeHaen, P. Science, Drugs, and the Food and Drug Administration. *New York State Journal of Medicine*, 1971, *71* (13).

Goldstein, A., Aronow, L., & Kalman, S. M. *Principles of Drug Action—The Basis of Pharmacology.* New York: Harper and Row, 1968.

Gutfreund, H. *An Introduction to the Study of Enzymes.* New York: Wiley, 1965.

Hartshorn, E. A., & Francke, D. E. Handbook of Drug Interactions. Ohio: 1970.

Hathaway, D. E. *Foreign Compound Metabolism in Mammals.* London: Chemical Society, 1970.

Jusko, W. J. Pharmacokinetic Principles in Pediatric Pharmacology. *Pediatric Clinics of North America*, 1972, *19* (1), 81-100.

LaDu, B. N. Pharmacogenetics: Defective Enzymes in Relation to Reaction to Drugs. *Annual Review of Medicine*, 1972, *23*, 453-468.

LaDu, B. N., & Kalow, W. Pharmacogenetics. *Annals of the New York Academy of Sciences*, 1968, *151*.

Notari, R. E. *Biopharmaceutics and Pharmacokinetics, an Introduction.* New York: Marcel Dekker, 1971.

Porter, C. C. *Chemical Mechanisms of Drug Action.* Springfield, Ill. Charles C. Thomas, 1970.

Roth, L. J. *Isotopes in Experimental Pharmacology.* Illinois: University of Chicago Press, 1965.

Shrader, S. R. *Introductory Mass Spectrometry.* Boston: Allyn & Bacon, 1971.

Steiner, R. F. *The Chemical Foundations of Molecular Biology.* New York: D. Van Nostrand, 1965.

Stockley, I. H. Basic Principles of Drug Interaction. *Chemistry in Britain*, 1972, *8*, 114-118.

Vessell, E. S. Drug Metabolism in Man. *Annals of the New York Academy of Sciences*, 1971, *179*.

Wagner, J. G. *Biopharmaceutics and Relevant Pharmacokinetics.* Hamilton, Illinois: Drug Intelligence Publications, 1971.

Wang, C. H. & Willis, D. L. *Radiotracer Methodology in Biological Science.* Englewood Cliffs, N.J.: Prentice-Hall, 1965.

Watson, J. D. *Molecular Biology of the Gene.* (2nd ed.) New York: W. A. Benjamin.

APPENDIX

Structural Formulas

It will be apparent to the reader of this volume that the medicinal chemist must have a means to describe the structures of the complex organic chemicals with which he works. In some of the chapters the structural features of the compounds are described to explain how the known drugs have been modified in the search for new ones with superior properties. In other chapters structural formulas of complex drugs are presented to describe their nature and complexity. It may be helpful to point out a few salient features in the graphic representation of structural formulas.

Figure 1 of Chapter 3 shows a space filling model of the morphine molecule placed beside a skeletal model of the same compound. It is customary to represent carbon atoms with black models, hydrogens with white, nitrogen with blue and oxygen with red. The three oxygen atoms stand out because each has only two bonds to adjacent atoms and, in the photograph has slots for forming hydrogen bonds. The nitrogen atom, with three bonds, is nearly surrounded with adjacent carbon atoms. In models without color, or in black and white photographs of models it is difficult to distinguish the nitrogen and carbon atoms, for each is often found at the junctions of three or four bonds. The hydrogen atoms, each with but a single bond, are easily visible at the corners of the skeletal model. In the space filling model some of the hydrogen atoms are hidden from our view by the other atoms closer to us.

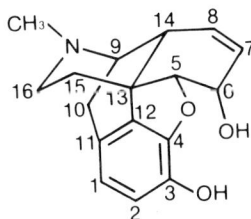

Morphine

The figure above is a structural formula showing the stereo-chemistry or shape of the morphine molecule in which the lines have the same meaning as in the skeletal model. Carbon atoms are understood to be located at the junctions of lines. If another atom, such as nitrogen or oxygen, is found there, the symbol for the hetero atom is used. The hydrogen atoms are omitted except for special circumstances such as when they are part of a methyl group (CH_3) or when attached to a hetero atom such as oxygen. Hydrogen atoms are joined to carbon atoms in the number and position required to complete the four valence bonds to carbon. Thus, at position 15, there are two hydrogen atoms. Similarly, at position 9 where the carbon atom is at the junction of three lines a hydrogen atom must be placed as illus-trated in the skeletal model. At position 13 where four lines meet there are no valence bonds left over and no hydrogens.

Another way in which the four valence bonds of carbon can be satisfied is the double bond such as between positions 7 and 8. Here only single atoms of hydrogen are required. These are visible in the skeletal model but are completely hidden in the view we have of the space filling model. The benzene ring is another special case. This planar ring of six carbon atoms is "aromatic" and only one valence bond is available for another atom at each of the six corners. If there is no carbon or hetero atom attached, it is assumed that a hydrogen atom is located at the corner position. Examples of compounds with aromatic rings are discussed in more detail in several of the chapters of this book.

Names of Drugs

Drugs taken by the patient are seldom single chemical entities. More often the active ingredient has been combined with some medically inert material and formulated into a tablet, a capsule or a solution. Individual manufacturers may formulate the same active ingredient in different ways and each resulting product may have its own characteristics. Especially important are biological availability and stability of the product. The names given by the manufacturers to their products are trade names and are usually different for each manufacturer even though the chemical identity of the active ingredient is the same in each case.

The active ingredients in medical practice are usually single chemical compounds. Each compound has a unique chemical structure and a definite chemical name. Rules for naming organic compounds have been established by the American Chemical Society and international rules have been laid down by the International Union of Pure and Applied Chemistry. It is apparent that the complexity of organic compounds often requires a complex chemical name.

Since these names are often very cumbersome to use, simplified names are usually employed. The trade names for drugs are proprietary names and are registered as trademarks in the United States Patent office. In order that useful nonproprietary names may be provided for new chemicals used as drugs the United States adopted names are coined by a council established for this purpose. This name is usually a single word of not more than four syllables which is simple and reflects pharmacologic, chemical or other characteristics and relationships of practical value to the users. U.S. adopted names have been used throughout this volume whenever possible to refer to the active moieties of the drugs described.

Receptor Theory

Numerous references have been made to drug-receptor sites which are believed to resemble the specificity cavities of enzymes. The frontispiece shows a Corey-Pauling-Koltun (CPK) space filling model of N-formyl-L-tryptophan in a skeletal model of the specificity cavity of the enzyme a-chymotrypsin. Atoms which line the surface of the cavity have CPK caps so that the model shows the close complementary fit between the virtual substrate molecule and the specificity cavity. The substrate is seen to be precisely positioned by a hydrogen bond between its amino group and a carbonyl oxygen atom at the entrance to the cavity. Model construction: Frank H. Clarke and Jeffrey W. H. Watthey; Photograph: Craig Cooper; Pharmaceuticals Division, CIBA-GEIGY Corporation.

THE AUTHORS

Dr. Mitchell N. Cayen was born in Montreal, Quebec, Canada and spent his undergraduate years at McGill and Cornell Universities. He received his B.Sc. and M.Sc. from McGill University in 1959 and 1961 respectively. In 1964 he received his Ph.D. in Biochemistry from McGill University. His Ph.D. thesis was concerned with the metabolism of plant estrogens. Dr. Cayen joined the Department of Biochemistry at Ayerst Research Laboratories in January, 1965, under a National Research Council of Canada grant to conduct basic studies on the pathogenesis of atherosclerosis. In 1968, he was appointed head of the newly formed Metabolism Section in charge of studies on lipid metabolism and drug metabolism.

Dr. Cayen's interests and responsibilities include the study of the metabolic fate of potential drugs in laboratory animals and man, and the control of lipid metabolism. He is the senior author of more than 30 publications.

Dr. Frank H. Clarke was born in Newcastle, New Brunswick, Canada. He received his B.Sc. and M.Sc. in Organic Chemistry from the University of New Brunswick in 1949 and 1950 respectively. In 1954 he received his Ph.D. in Organic Chemistry from Harvard University. After two years of post-doctorate research at Columbia University he joined the Medicinal Chemistry Department of Schering Corporation where he became Senior Research Chemist in 1959. He joined Geigy Chemical Corporation in 1962 where he was appointed Director of Medicinal Chemistry in 1967. In this position he was responsible for the Departments of Organic Chemistry, Biochemistry and Molecular Biology and for the Kilo Laboratory. He is presently Deputy Director of the Chemistry Division in the Research Department of the Pharmaceuticals Division, CIBA-GEIGY Corporation.

169

Dr. Clarke's publications are mainly in the areas of the synthesis of natural products and of potential medicinal agents. His interests include the use of drug metabolism in the design of new medicinal agents and the study of enzymes as models for pharmacological receptor sites.

Dr. George deStevens was born in Tarrytown, New York. He received his Ph.D. in organic chemistry from Fordham University in 1953. The title of his thesis was "The Chemistry of Lignin and Biochemical Implications of this substance in Woody Tissues". This work was carried out under the mentorship of Professor F. F. Nord. Dr. deStevens joined CIBA Pharmaceutical Company in 1955 as a senior chemist and was promoted to Director of Medicinal Chemistry in 1961. He became Director of Chemical Research in 1966 and in June 1967 was promoted to Vice President and Director of Research. He is presently Executive Vice President and Director of Research of the Pharmaceuticals Division, CIBA-GEIGY Corporation.

Dr. deStevens has authored and co-authored approximately 100 scientific papers and holds 65 patents in the area of medicinal chemistry. He is the author of a book on diuretics and editor of another volume on analgetics. Dr. deStevens is also editor of a series of monographs on Medicinal Chemistry.

Dr. Hershel L. Herzog, a native of New York City, received his professional education at the University of Illinois (B.Sc. in Chemical Engineering, summa cum laude) and the University of Southern California (M.Sc., Ph.D—organic chemistry). He has spent substantially the whole of his career as laboratory worker and manager with the Schering Corporation, a New Jersey pharmaceutical firm, whose employ he entered in 1950. At present he holds the position of Director of Chemical Research and Development.

Dr. Herzog's principal research interests have been in steroid hormones and antibiotics, and more generally in the applications of microorganisms to the discovery and development of drugs. He is the co-author of a handbook "Microbiological Transformation of Steroids" and about 50 articles concerned with various aspects of organic chemistry. Dr. Herzog has been prominently associated with two major drug discoveries, the prednisone family of anti-inflammatory steroid hormones and gentamicin, an antibiotic now widely used to treat serious gram-negative infections.

Dr. Gordon E. Mallett was born in Lafayette, Indiana, and went to school in Evansville, Indiana. He received a B.Sc. in Chemistry at Purdue in 1949, and his Ph.D. in Microbiology at Purdue in 1956. After completing his training he was employed at Fort Detrick for one year with the U. S. Army Biological Laboratories. In 1957 he accepted a position with Eli Lilly and Company in the Microbiological Research Department. He worked in various assignments, exploring the chemical activities of microorganisms.

Dr. Mallett was involved in research on the semi-synthetic penicillins and cephalosporins, developing a wide interest in both chemical and microbiological aspects of antibiotic research. In 1966 he was made Head, and in 1968, Director of the Fermentation Products Research Division. At present he is Director of Research, Lilly Research Centre, Windlesham, Surrey, England.

Dr. William M. McLamore was born in Shreveport, Louisiana. He received B.A. and M.A. degrees from Rice Institute in 1941 and 1943 respectively, and the Ph.D. degree in organic chemistry from Harvard University in 1949. He joined Pfizer Inc. in 1950. He was appointed Section Manager in 1961, and he is presently engaged in Research Administration. Dr. McLamore's contributions to medicinal chemistry include drug discoveries in the areas of hypnotics sedatives (ethchlorvynol), sulfonylurea anti-diabetic drugs (chlorpropamide) and thiazide diuretics (benzthiazide).

Dr. Albert J. Plummer was born in Somerville, Massachusetts. He received his A.B. and A.M. degrees from Boston University and also his Ph.D. in Biochemistry. His M.D. was obtained from the Boston University School of Medicine. From 1935 until

1949 he was engaged in teaching and research in pharmacology at the Boston University School of Medicine, where he was an Associate Professor.

Since 1949 Dr. Plummer has been associated with the Biology Division at CIBA-GEIGY Corporation in Summit, New Jersey, where, until May 1, 1973, he was Executive Director of Biological Research. He is now Consultant to Biological Research. His research interests have been primarily in the field of antihypertensive drugs, cardiovascular drugs, diuretics and compounds acting on the central nervous system.

Dr. Naokata Yokoyama is a Senior Staff Scientist in the Pharmaceuticals Division of CIBA-GEIGY Corporation. He was born in Osaka, Japan in 1933. After receiving his B.Sc. and M.Sc. degrees from Osaka University in 1956 and 1958 respectively, he attended the University of Wisconsin and received his Ph.D. degree in Pharmaceutical Chemistry in 1963. His research activities at Osaka and Wisconsin Universities resulted in several publications in the field of alkaloid chemistry. He joined the Medicinal Chemistry Department of Geigy Chemical Corporation in 1963, where he became a Project Leader, responsible for the development of analgesic agents.

Dr. Charles L. Zirkle is Associate Director of Chemistry at the Research Laboratories of Smith Kline and French Laboratories, Philadelphia, Pennsylvania. After obtaining a B.Sc. in chemistry from Indiana University in 1942, he worked three years in the chemistry laboratories of Smith Kline and French. Dr. Zirkle then entered the University of Illinois where he received a Ph.D. in organic chemistry in 1949. Since rejoining the company he has done research in several fields of medicinal chemistry. Over the past 12 years Dr. Zirkle's primary research interests have been the synthesis and chemistry of psychopharmacological agents.

Index

Abel, J. J., 103
absorption, 140, 143, 157
acetanilide, 31
acetazolamide, 45, 47, 159
acetohexamide, 47
acetophenetidine, 31
acetylcholine, 39, 110, 113, 117, 119
addiction liability, 30
Addison, William, 95
adrenal gland, 82
adrenocorticotrophic hormone (ACTH), 103
agar plate, 17
Ahlquist, R. P., 115
albumin, 135, 157
Allen, W. M., 92
allopurinol, 137
alpha blockers, 118
alphamethyldopa, 126
alphamethylmetatyrosine, 126
alphamethylnorepinephrine, 126
alphamethylparatyrosine, 126
alpha receptors, 115, 116
6-aminopenicillanic acid, 22
amitriptyline, 70
analgesics, 29
angiotensin, 120
antibiotics, 13
antibodies, 136, 161
antidepressant, 71
antidepressives, 70
antidiabetic, 46
antihistamines, 3, 62, 69
antihypertensive agents, 51
antipsychotic, 57, 67, 68, 71
antipyretic, 31
antipyrine, 161
antitussive, 31, 36

apomorphine, 64
Archer, Sydney, 37
arterioles, 83
arteriosclerosis, 107
Aschheim, S., 90
aspirin, 31, 141, 158
ataraxics, 57
atrophine, 33
autoradiography, 145

Banting, Frederick, 102
barium chloride, 120
baroceptors, 113
Bayliss, Sir William Maddock, 101, 102
Beecher, Henry, 36
Bein, Hugo, 121
Bergman, W., 96
Bernthsen, A., 59
Berthold, 86, 90
Best, Charles, 102
beta receptors, 115
bethanidine, 124
Beyer, Karl, 47, 48, 49
biochemical rationale, 138
biopharmaceutics, 141
biopolymers, 133
biotransformation, 149
blocker (alpha or beta), 115
blood-brain barrier, 145
blood pressure, 107
Bovet, D., 62
Brodie, Bernard, 148
bronchioles, 83
Butenandt, Adolph, 88

carbonic anhydrase, 45, 50
carbutamide, 46
Carlsson, Arvid, 122

173